Aquarian-Age Healing

Bio-Mechanics

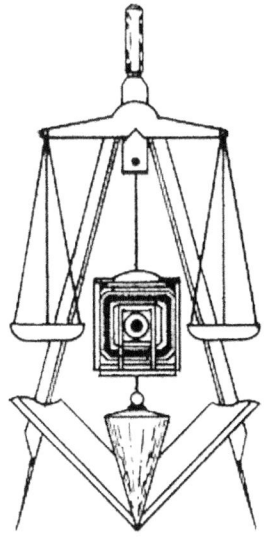

John Hurley, D.C., and Helen Sanders, D.C., Ph.C.

Reformatted, lightly edited, and
comprehensively indexed
by
Ken Ladd and Shay O'Neal

Foreword by Ken Ladd

Cg Publishing

Aquarian-Age Healing
Bio-Mechanics
Book One

Hurley and Sanders
Original publication 1932
Appendix publication 1936
Los Angeles, California USA

ISBN 978-0-69247-667-3

Cg Publishing
Jasper, Arkansas USA

Cover photograph by Ben Ostrowsky
  Foucault's Pendulum, taken at the Museo Nazionale della Scienza e della Tecnologia Leonardo da Vinci (Leonardo da Vinci National Museum of Science and Technology) in Milan, Italy, June 1996.

Cover design by Kyley "Sharpie" Sturgeon

Interior illustrations by Raymond C. McIntyre

Printed in the United States of America

www.aquarianagehealing.com

Dedicated to the memory of
Dr. John H. Tomlinson

Table of Contents

FOREWORD

Holding one hand on a spot on my abdomen and the other hand directly opposite on my back, I asked Doc, "Do you think these two painful spots could be related to each other?" He gave me a long quizzical look before answering, "Of course they're related." I felt a relief upon hearing these words that was almost an epiphany, not because his answer surprised me but because it validated exactly what I was feeling and what my logic was telling me. It was important because during the months leading up to this moment, I had asked several medical doctors, including a surgeon who specialized in internal medicine, this same question, and each had answered, "No, I don't see any relationship," and said that each spot should be treated by a different specialist. On the other hand, Doc viewed the body as a whole, each part dependent on all other parts for maximum health and function. He was surprised I asked.

Dr. (Doc) John H. Tomlinson used a treatment he called Bio-Mechanics, which consisted of a plumb-line analysis of posture, or distortion, followed by a light-touch protocol on a therapy table. After two sessions of approximately twenty minutes each, I was completely out of pain (including both spots), and the pain never returned.

Thus began a nearly thirty-year ongoing journey of exploration into the principles of healthy living, starting with classes in Bio-Mechanics and Bio-Engineering taught by Doc's contemporary, Dr. E.F. Hayles. During the 1940s, they had been students of Dr. John L. Hurley, who had developed a system of healing called Aquarian-Age Healing.

Dr. Hurley and Dr. Helen Sanders, Hurley's wife and business partner for about six years, co-authored two books: *Aquarian-Age Healing for You* (Book One), written for lay people and published in 1932; and *Aquarian-Age Healing: Bio-Engineering* (Book Two), written for professionals and published in 1933. Hurley and Sanders gave lectures and taught seminars in the United States and abroad during the early 1930s. In 1936 they published a thirty-page pamphlet that updated the original *Book One* technic chapter with more detailed instructions, more specific application procedures, and revisions to several steps in the original procedure. This pamphlet was included at the end of later printings of *Book One* as an appendix. The updated *Book One* was retitled *Aquarian-Age Healing: Bio-Mechanics*. It is this later book that is represented in this publication, which preserves all of the material and concepts of the original *Book One* plus the revisions and updates of the *Appendix*.

Book One was written for lay people because the authors believed that there were several fundamental and simple ways to prevent disease or recover from disease and injury by following procedures that were easy for the average person to learn and apply. The book was published at a time of conflict and change among chiropractors, osteopaths, pharmacists, medical doctors, and others. The theory and method of healing that it describes differed from all other approaches. It was named *Aquarian-Age Healing* because in that coming age it was prophesied that a person would be his brother's keeper, and the authors envisioned that *Book One* would enable ordinary people to help each other.

Dr. Hayles and Dr. Tomlinson considered that the original theories and the development of application technics were the work of John Hurley and that contributions by Helen Sanders were mainly in the areas of experimentation and confirmation. After Hurley and Sanders divorced and dissolved their working relationship in 1937, Dr. Sanders continued her own career and made a lasting contribution to the chiropractic field.

Dr. Hurley's originality of thinking resulted from his experience as a mechanical engineer and as a chiropractor. His combined knowledge, applied over a span of fifteen years of research, culminated in the ideas presented in *Book One* and *Book Two*. He viewed human physiology, from the neuromusculoskeletal system down to the cellular level, through the lens of Newtonian physics. He understood the importance of environmental influences on the structure and functioning of the human body, and he recognized disease processes in terms of degrees of fatigue.

Dr. Hurley originated the terms *Bio-Mechanics* and *Bio-Engineering* to describe his technics.[1] He was the first person to use the term *stress*, as an engineering concept, to describe the body's normal and healthy reaction to various environmental forces, predating Hans Selye's very different and complex use of the term by several years. Hurley's main focus was on *distortion*, its causes, its effects, and the means for its correction. The subjects covered in *Book One* include stress, strain, distortion, adaptation, fatigue, disease, acidosis, and exhaustion. Gentle technics are introduced that use very simple tools to rebalance the body around its center of gravity, relieve strain, and promote rest and a return to homeostasis.

---

[1] The earliest combination of *bio* and *mechanics* has been attributed to contemporaries of Dr. Hurley in Russia. Vsevolod Meyerhold and N.A. Bernstein separately used the term *biomekhanika* beginning in the 1920s, about the same time Hurley was developing his own theories. As generalized terms, *biomechanics* and *bio-engineering* came into more common usage in the second half of the twentieth century.

Book One may seem to overstate certain ideas. For example, it states that any pain can be controlled immediately by the proper application of Bio-Mechanics technic and that every disease can be successfully resolved by following the procedures outlined in the book. Logic will suggest that this is not likely to always be the case. A careful reading, however, reveals that the authors *were* realistic about the healing process, stating that in cases of long-standing injury or disease the body needs time to rebuild itself and that no one can get function from destroyed organs. There is a progression of disease (expressed as *fatigue*) from mild symptoms like soreness all the way to atrophy, degeneration, and death. Disease becomes increasingly difficult to reverse in its later stages; and after severe injury or disease, or invasive medical or surgical interventions, the organism can reach a stage of alteration that is beyond its ability to recover its previous normal function. *Book One* also seems to overstress the dangers inherent in wrong application of technic. Dr. Hurley's further research and development led to lighter inputs and pressures as well as simplified technics, which made application procedures very safe to learn and use. His classes included cautions and contraindications to be considered in working with any person.

The authors state that Aquarian-Age Healing opens immense new fields of discovery in areas needing further investigation. It was Dr. Hurley's hope that people would use his ideas and discover ways to reverse *all* diseases and injuries using simple, natural technics, and that his technics would become a common tool in the prevention of, or early intervention in, most diseases and injuries.

Book One was the early development of Bio-Mechanics, not the finished procedure. Throughout Dr. Hurley's career, he continued to develop and improve his ideas and methods. The *Appendix* published in 1936 updated and clarified the technic information in the original *Book One*, but the numerous and important revisions made after 1936 were never published.

Dr. Hurley stated in 1942 that, while his fundamental principles and objectives remained the same as when discovered and published, his instruction, lectures, and technic were constantly being clarified and developed and that his latest ideas and procedures were always taught in his seminars.

Dr. Hurley's unpublished ideas and technics were preserved by several of his last students, including Dr. Tomlinson and Dr. Hayles, both of whom attended Dr. Hurley's last classes from 1945 to 1947. Dr. Hayles repeated the class five times during this period and was able to record Dr. Hurley's entire classroom lectures verbatim by taking notes in his own shorthand. His notes are believed to be the final version of Dr. Hurley's seminars.

Dr. Hurley's latest developments and revisions are not included in this publication of *Book One* because they evolved over time to such an extent that they cannot be incorporated without major change to the book. The purpose of the present publication is to preserve Dr. Hurley's original ideas and to follow the progression of his thinking through his own writings. The original text has been minimally edited for readability, and the only additions are the following:

1. "notes" and numbered footnotes for informational purposes,

2. a glossary containing Dr. Hurley's later definitions of concepts used in the book,

3. the current "Foreword;" the original "Foreword" has been renamed "Preface," and

4. a comprehensive index for easy access to all subjects.

In addition to its value as a resource for Dr. Hurley's followers, the current publication serves the purpose of introducing *Aquarian-Age Healing: Bio-Mechanics* to a new audience, providing insight into many areas of wellness and disease. Chapter XVII and the Appendix give valuable information as to how the technic works, though these early procedural instructions should not be used for therapeutic application due to the reasons given above.

Aquarian-Age Healing: Bio-Engineering (Book Two) is in final form for publication. *Book Two* gives much more comprehensive treatment to subjects such as anatomy and physiology, chemical and electrical balances, colloid chemistry, the importance of posture as an indicator of health, the adaptation process involved in health degradation, the functioning of the body in its environment, and the disease process. It introduces several potent technics for gently working with the body to help reverse more complex adaptational patterns. Though *Book Two* was originally published for professionals, Dr. Hurley later devised methods for simplifying the instruction to include the serious lay person. Drawing upon contemporary knowledge and research, Dr. Hurley completes and validates his theories on health and disease processes in *Book Two*.

The release of *Book Two* will be followed by a future book based on Dr. Hurley's latest teachings. This book will preserve Dr. Hurley's final ideas and technics and will include my own experiences, results, and observations using this work for the past three decades.

Aquarian-Age Healing: Bio-Mechanics suggests that in seeking a healthy lifestyle we use preventive methods and simple, natural remedies whenever possible. Extraordinary measures such as medicines and surgery, though sometimes necessary for the preservation of life, add complexity to the disease process that may alter the organism to such an extent that complete recovery is difficult. A true reversal of disease or injury is more beneficial than altering the body through complex interventions. This book gives important insights into how the body functions, with health, restoration, and longevity as its goals.

Ken Ladd
2015, Jasper Arkansas

PREFACE

What is Aquarian-Age Healing? Why is it so named?

Aquarian-Age Healing is a science, an art, and a philosophy of life and living which presents a rational, mechanical, scientific, and more or less skilled art of analysis of all things abnormal, more especially as applied to human ills, and a philosophy of doing and being which is so simple and free from complexity as to be comprehensible to the savage and at the same time to intrigue and interest the most highly trained special scientist in the corrections following such analyses.

It is named Healing because by its radical departure from all previous teachings it becomes healing in actuality instead of merely attempted and sometimes palliative treatment.

It is named Aquarian-Age because its advent could only occur in the beginning years of that Golden Age of prophecy, and because it is one of the most important of a large number of revolutionary changes that must occur before all the prophecies of this age can be realized.

We find, in relation to this, statements in many places in the Bible that, during the period when the constellation of Aquarius (the water-bearer, the son of man) occupies the eastern horizon, mankind will realize the brotherhood of man;

that all honor will be paid to the man of honor (instead of to the dishonorables who happen to be in power or to be immensely wealthy) and that consequently government will become honest, as men will be; that due to this there shall be no more wars and no more crime; that there shall no more be sorrow, pain, tears, and death; that man shall make the last conquest of the material and ultimately turn his eyes with singleness of purpose to the spiritual. Such statements are found in all sacred writings in such abundance that we believe there is a true and solid foundation for them, and that since the constellation of Aquarius is now rising, the beginning of the realization of these prophecies can now be expected.

We know that now for the first time in history it is possible to point out so clearly and teach so simply what causes pain and disease and how to ameliorate them that the average layman can learn the art without trouble and apply his knowledge successfully. Whether or not the ancient prophecies are due to be realized, this art did require a new name, and as no other seemed competent, this was adopted.

It may be interesting to point out that at the dawn of history the constellation of Gemini was occupying the same position in the sky, and we find everything in pairs, as Adam and Eve, Cain and Abel, and at the close of this age, Noah took on the Ark all his offspring and all animals in pairs. Then the constellation of Taurus (the Bull) took its place, and the Bull was used for sacrifice, and strength and endurance without great intelligence or sensitiveness was the ordinary criterion of greatness. Moses led the Jews out of Egypt at the time when the Taurian Age was being replaced by the Arian Age (the Ram), and we find that in order to avoid one phase of the plague, they had to sprinkle their lintels with the blood of the lamb. Yet when they had wandered in the wilderness, they lapsed back into the Taurian Age when they again returned to the worship of the calf. In the Arian Age, the ram or sheep supplanted the bull as a sacrifice, and resignation and an unquestioning "follow the leader" idea was considered the mark of rectitude.

This age was followed by the Piscean Age (Fish) when the constellation of that name was on the ascendant and the identification of the early Christian was made possible by the mark of the fish. Though Jesus was the Lamb of God, still he taught his disciples to be fishers of men, for that period was another transition period. Now, the constellation of Aquarius is displacing Pisces, and if history repeats itself, changes may be expected in the next few centuries equivalent to those that occurred in the early years of previous rising constellations. Each of these periods occupies a little over two thousand years.

However that may be, the work we teach has the merit that should admit it to that distinguished company, if such does exist, and we ourselves are confident that we have not misnamed it nor appropriated a name that is undeserved.

One of the reasons for this attitude is that for ourselves we ask nothing except the privilege of continued activity. A study of this work will disclose many points demanding further research. We have publicly dedicated our lives to the continued research that will further increase the comfort and happiness of the human race, both mental and physical.

As in any new idea and method, we are met with questionings and suspicions at every turn. For a period of two years, both in Europe and in America, we have earnestly endeavored to get this work to suffering humanity through the medium of public institutions. We have been met with some courtesy and little interest. To date, all persons who have given us audience have admitted we have a common-sense, practical, and logical explanation of the cause of disease and a simple, understandable method for its correction; yet we have never been permitted to demonstrate in any clinic under authoritative observation and checking. We offered to demonstrate the efficiency of our work in cancer cases to an eminent cancer specialist of San Francisco,* promising to show relief from pain and a general improvement in any case or cases of his own choosing. An appointment was made for such demonstrations, but the doctor was called out of town, and we have heard nothing from him since, and that was November 1930. This is merely one instance, which has repeated itself in Europe.

However, we are undaunted and will continue pioneering in our mission of eliminating pain and disease from this earth and enlightening mankind, as has been promised to this age, being convinced that truth will prevail.

---

* The publishers of this book will be glad to furnish the physician's name upon request. [Note: Information is no longer available.]

INTRODUCTION

There are three major causes of unhappiness. In their order they are:

Pain and Dis-ease

Want

Thwarted Ambition

The contents of this book will remove from the life of every person who masters it all fear of pain and disease, the primal and most potent cause of unhappiness, because when in pain or ill, even want loses its bite and ambitions are forgotten.

This book is written for the layman. We believe, and we hope the belief will prove to be well-founded, that any person who will take this book, read, then study its contents, perform the routine necessary, carefully, accurately, and exactly in accord with the directions given, will find himself able to perform all we promise. That promise is that the method herein taught will INSTANTLY STOP ANY PAIN. And if the routine presented is persistently followed will ultimately cure any disease.

This routine requires time and effort to master. There is no magic formula. There is no mysterious "control." There is nothing but a reasonable, logical, practical method for doing the thing the body requires to have done when it is sick to bring it back to health, and the results are instant, positive, and dependable IN EVERY CASE, and any man who will follow instructions can secure these results.

This book represents an important departure from usual methods. Its theory and philosophy strike at the roots of important interests. The whole practice of medicine, to say nothing of groups of lesser importance, will be seriously affected if and when the procedures herein laid down come into general use. Methods of caring for those ill, methods of determining what care they require, and all the agencies employed will, upon realizing the import of this work, undoubtedly use all means to prevent its general acceptance, and in this endeavor they will most likely have the active support of the "critic."

The "critics" have apparently committed themselves to the idea that only those who forward the *aesthetic* development of humanity and those who contribute directly thereto are important, essential, or entitled to any large financial returns for their efforts. To this "advanced class" belong by admission of the critics themselves, most artists, most actors, most writers of fiction and poetry, and of course practically all critics. The scientist upon whose work all the foundation of our present advance is laid must, however, according to Mr. Llewellyn Jones in his book, *How to Criticize Books*, take his findings to his superiors or groups of inferiors and there see his work mutilated or destroyed, or perhaps occasionally accepted, without expecting or receiving any remuneration beyond the actual cost of disseminating his new knowledge.

Such a situation is unfair and, except in a certain frame of mind, dishonest. We do not believe Mr. Jones is dishonest; therefore let us try to find his state of mind and the reasons for it. We use Mr. Jones as an illustration because he is one of the foremost American critics and, as such, one of the "leaders of American thought." He is the author of many serious books, editor of the Chicago Evening Post, a contributor to the Northwestern University "The New World Series," and altogether a man of intelligence whose opinions are sought and valued by numbers of people.

Now to illustrate our point, and because we expect our work will draw plenty of adverse criticism from these "critics," we quote Mr. Jones from the book above mentioned.

"But suppose we meet somebody who tells us that a great teacher has arisen who has discovered a new law governing human life – it might be 'the law of the octave' which is the latest thing to come to my attention and that through the utilization of his law we can increase our mental and spiritual stature a cubit or so? What shall be our criterion? I have a simple and infallible criterion that anybody can apply.... Then ask: how much does it cost to learn this new truth? In the case of 'the law of the octave' it was ten dollars for four weekly lectures or two and a half dollars at the door as you entered for each lecture. And I immediately knew that this law was nonsense.

"This does not mean that I was shy the $2.50 – not any more than I usually am, that is – and it does not mean that I am making fun of the idea. I mean this seriously and literally; any idea that is urged upon your attention with the suggestion that you pay for learning about it is false – and false either for the reason that its initiator is a fakir or is a lunatic. For real knowledge is always recognized by two characteristics: It is communistic and it is never pushed by propaganda...."

Communism is a hateful word according to other writings by the same author. Nothing good can be expected of anything communistic; his tirade against Sinclair Lewis upon the award of the Nobel Prize in 1930 is evidence enough of this, yet *knowledge must be communistic*. Mr. Jones also says in the same book, "Nobody knows today how much our communications of written or spoken words, outside of sheer sensationalism [that is] characteristic of our press, is propaganda for special interest." He also mentions that Professor John Dewey has written a book entitled *The Public and Its Problems*, and most highly recommends it to the public. He says this book offers the best and only practical solution for the abuses of predatory – special – interest, and commits himself to its method. That method is one of education of the masses as to their obligations to maintain the integrity of the government. In view of this statement just quoted relating to propaganda (which exists in its most unadulterated form in our public schools), the methods outlined of securing this education and having the masses benefit therefrom seems rather puerile. But that is not the main point. The remedies are aimed at *existing conditions*. The author, Professor Dewey, admits that a generation or two at least will be needed to bring his program to effectiveness and he apparently expects these "special interests" to sit quietly by and remain in a defenseless state during all of the time the masses are preparing themselves to annihilate these interests. We know positively from all the experience of the people of the whole world that nothing of that sort will happen. And the reason it will not happen is that knowledge must be communistic – knowledge alone.

This means that all new knowledge, according to Mr. Jones, must be given gratis, if it be true knowledge, to all who want it. But the masses of people have no means of using it or profiting by it except through their government. Only "special interest" is in a position, by means of special organization, to fit it into any large program, and consequently such programs grow, develop, and become ever more menacing to the masses by this very fact.

Special interest is a manifestation of selfishness, which reaches a point of disregard of the rights of others. The government of the United States, in theory at least, regards the rights of all against the encroachment of these selfish purposes and hence the conflict is fundamental, never ending unless or until other goals than power and money can be substituted for these.

What means does special interest use? Every means conceivable by the best brains to be had. How are such services secured? By the creation of the ideas in the minds of the "critic" that knowledge alone must be communistic and that endowments, gifts, and other prerequisites, representing only small parts of the plunder of special interests, sufficiently repay the masses for the things stolen. By the last they secure the first; thence it is carried to the masses themselves by propaganda, decried by these very folk through the press, the movie, the radio, and the public school, and by them, through controlled elections in which fundamental questions are never raised, back to the government, now complacent and regardless of the rights of the masses because those very masses have in their elections approved the activities of these predatory interests and the "Intelligencia." The critics are the greatest single factor in the operation, even though they themselves are unconscious of their part in it, as we believe Mr. Jones to be.

So that while none of those close to us believe we are "lunatics" and any honest test, which we welcome, will prove we are not "fakirs," still we feel we are entitled to a price for our work. And also in addition, we are ourselves committed to the use of such resources as may develop for the closing of such gaps as still exist in the group of facts essential to our argument.

There is another group of people, true scientists, who will, we hope, take the material herein offered and prove that which is true, improve that which we only can offer and make usable to the average man, the tremendous values of which we can prove by demonstration to be inherent in it.

When this is undertaken, every bit of development that occurs under such a program will raise the average of happiness and ease among the masses of people far more than any other single thing that could be accomplished. To this group we offer our work. Then will be found some very significant facts. The arguments are impossible at this time to complete, only, we believe, because colloid chemistry and allied science has not yet developed the facts we need to make our position bullet-proof.

"It is not the falling stick that leaves its mark upon the minds and hearts of men, nor leaves its imprint upon their consciousness.

"It is the LIGHT the rocket sheds upon the world during its brief career and especially that which marked its highest flight and its best accomplishment.

"It will suit me and satisfy me if my life can be so spent, can so end and be so forgotten, because there is no more reason to preserve or remember the body that once carried the 'Me' than to preserve or remember the stick that once carried the rocket."

J. Hurley

CHAPTER I...THE HUMAN EQUATION

The entire practice of medicine or any therapy depends first on correct diagnosis. Any medical doctor will tell you that before any hope of improvement in your trouble can be entertained, a correct diagnosis must be made because treatment is directed by the information thus derived. Just as an illustration (enough are available to fill this book), treatment for appendicitis differs greatly from treatment for gallstones, and treatment for gallstones differs greatly from that required in a case of pneumonia; so that successful outcome as in those cases that recover depends upon the adoption of the treatment for the true trouble. The treatment for gallstones would be entirely wrong and damage a patient who was in fact suffering from pneumonia or appendicitis, and so it can be seen that a correct diagnosis really is of prime importance.

But these diseases are often mistaken each for the other, and the error is not discovered until and unless death occurs and the body is subjected to an autopsy. This statement would be unbelievable if there were no other grounds for it than the opinion of the authors. But there are other grounds for it, viz: the authority of Dr. Cabot of Massachusetts General Hospital, who is probably the highest medical authority in the United States today and who is Professor of Internal Medicine at Harvard University, one of the best, if not the best, medical colleges in America. He says that of all the cases in that hospital over a period of many years that died and went to autopsy, only 48% were correctly diagnosed. That is, the other 52% were treated for diseases they did not have, and these cases cover all sorts of conditions.

Even the commonest and supposedly most easily recognized diseases showed an appalling percentage of errors, indicating that, had those mistakes *not* been made, many of these cases could have been reasonably expected to recover because effective treatment for the disease was well known.

This is the performance in the very best hospital with the best of brains and material equipment possible to obtain, and the place where an intensive effort is made and has been consistently made over a long period of time to improve that average, yet almost wholly without changing the original percentages. When following the wrong path, one never arrives at the goal.

Reflect for a moment. If this really is true, and we would not dare print it if it were false, if over one-half (52% at our last information) of diagnoses made under the above conditions are wrong, what are the probable percentages in ordinary illnesses, where the physician is called upon to take a temperature, feel a pulse, look at a tongue, take in whatever else he can see, ask a few questions, and prescribe a treatment. The mind will automatically reply, "This cannot be so, no matter who makes the statement, because of all the people I know who go to a physician when they get sick, most of them get well and only those die who could not be saved." The answer to this divides itself into several ideas as follows:

First – All the contagious and infectious diseases are described in the text-books taught in the classrooms and known by experience to be "self-limiting" diseases. That is, they have a well-defined period of "incubation" during which the patient is gradually becoming ill; they become sufficiently ill to demand help and attention; they reach a climax or critical period; the patient passes the crisis and dies or recovers.

This is the course, and it does not matter at all whether any treatment or none is instituted, the disease will follow this course. A correct diagnosis and a proper treatment will help the patient. Proper methods will assist in passing the crisis and will greatly minimize and sometimes completely control any bad after-effects, "sequelae." But no *treatment* will change the typical history of that disease. Our teaching, being a *correction* of underlying trouble, does change the history of the disease, and *at once*. This is the difference.

If no error is made by the medical doctor, if everything done from the beginning to the end is exactly adapted to the patient, if a number of other obscure factors which are now beginning to be understood are all used to the best advantage, the patient makes a rapid and complete recovery, is said to have had a "light attack" and the doctor gets little credit. Whereas, if the doctor is "not so good," fails to recognize the condition at once or its full import, merely treats symptoms as they arise, does not know how to bring into the picture all the reserve and vital forces of the patient at a time when they can be effectively used, but permits these forces to lie dormant and be exhausted by the ravages of the disease, the patient becomes ever more ill, and recovers, if at all, only after a long struggle and usually with very definite and disastrous after-effects. In this case, the doctor is usually credited with being a wonderful fellow, with "pulling his patient through a terrible illness," and is credited with a wonderful cure – to all of which he is no more entitled than is the garage man entitled to be regarded as good, who tears your whole automobile apart and returns to you a disabled car when only the carburetor needed adjustment. He may tell you that he put in new pistons, rings, etc., and he may have made a good job of that, but if all of this was unnecessary, he either is no mechanic or he is not working in your interest. He is dealing with a material possession that you can duplicate if you must, whereas the doctor is dealing with your comfort and happiness and that of those around you. Yes, even with your very life.

Second – After such diseases have passed, there are, *as a rule*, sequelae left in their train, and sometimes these are so serious as to be as great a threat against life and frequently, as just pointed out, almost as great a threat against happiness and effectiveness as the disease itself. This may be seen in the frequent inability to walk after infantile paralysis. No such after-effects will ever be left if the disease is properly handled and cleared up. The basis for this statement is found in the experience with methods exactly adapted for the care of such disease, the one we teach for example, and in the fact that this work will clear the body of all such after-effects even when of years and years standing.

Third – All chronic diseases have their origin in such beginnings – acute diseases incompletely cured. This is a matter not susceptible of complete proof, but the facts are observed so frequently, so uniformly do people under non-medical care report this history, and so uniformly do they respond to the technic herein taught, that we have no fear of successful attack either on the theoretical or practical grounds. The theoretical basis for this statement will appear upon further perusal of this volume. It is in these people, as life approaches and passes the thirtieth year, that the effects of the aborted and suppressed diseases of childhood herein discussed commence to rob the person of comfort and effectiveness. They become unable to carry on as before and are unaccountably tired; they lose the springiness, elasticity, and drive that they should have, and they attribute their troubles to the immediate symptom most prominent *at the time*. Constipation usually exists, headaches, neuralgias, more or less pain in the back, legs, abdomen, neck, etc.; they take pills, powders, pain killers, and so on. Then they manage to have an operation or two, thus constantly going from bad to worse until by the time they are sixty they are old, they know it, and they commence to get ready to die.

We believe this is entirely wrong, unnecessary, and not at all what should be at the age of sixty. We believe it because we see these people change from such states back to full effectiveness again under the technic taught, and they do it regularly. This is one of the points of greatest importance in the work we teach — its *unfailing results.* Now, the next question will be, "Why is correct diagnosis so difficult?" and again we must separate our reply into a number of parts.

First — Because physiology, that is, the study of the functions of the body and its various parts during health and, therefore, the first fundamental requirement in recognizing a departure therefrom in disease, is largely unknown or incorrectly known. Here again is a statement unbelievable on our authority alone because physiology is one of the standard subjects even in the public schools and is taught each day as though it were merely a group of well-known and completely established facts, unchanging and permanent, in spite of the fact that the very next day it may be different because proven untrue.

For instance, the lungs take in and give out air, and during the period the air remains in the lungs there is an exchange of carbon dioxide for oxygen, and this interchange is necessary to life. But other substances have been found in the air besides oxygen. What does the lung do with these other substances? No physiology gives the answer. Yet we know, as noted in our chapter on the ductless glands, that dilution of materials to such a point that the original substances are infinitesimal are "activating principles" of some of our most necessary functions. For instance, the lack of growth or excessive growth, lack of function or an excess of it can be traced directly and positively to these minute principles. Is it impossible that some of the infinitely dilute or tenuous properties of our atmosphere, just now being discovered or not even discovered yet, may have tremendous effect on our bodies? And if this should prove true, then would not our physiologies again have to be rewritten in the chapters on the function of breathing and all thereto related? Certainly.

Exactly this has happened, not especially in relation to the lungs, but generally; is now happening and must continue to happen, for no knowledge is complete on earth today. No Truth is Absolute and no science can be completely scientific until all science is complete and absolute Truth is known. Therefore it will be understood that nothing in this work is meant to discredit, destroy, or minimize in any way any of the accomplishments of any school of treatment or healing or any of our scientific advances. But there is another angle as discussed in Chapters XIII and XIV which is necessary, however, in order to bring the public mind and the mind of the reader back to the true state of affairs from which most lay and some professional minds have been deliberately led away by the propaganda of organized political medicine. But now let us go on with our physiology.

Einstein is reported to have said something to the effect that weather reports would never be of any real value until a change identical with that which occurred when "Astrology became astronomy, changed meteorology into meteoronomy," -ology to -onomy, significant endings.*

And we have today physiology, not "physionomy," the result being that changes in fundamental subjects are constantly being made in physiology. We quote from the preface of *Kirke's Handbook of Physiology, Twenty-First Edition,* which is a standard textbook and used in practically every English-speaking school that teaches anything in relation to the care of the sick. It is recognized as an authority and quoted in other

---

* In the naming of this work, the reader will note that astronomy has been considered along with astrology and occult teachings, including the Bible. There are some beliefs contained in -ologies that are proven by their -onomies. As our knowledge increases, all -ologies will become -onomies.

standard textbooks. "The rapid progress that Physiology has made within the last few years has necessitated somewhat extensive alterations in the present edition. The chapters dealing with the proteins, blood coagulation, digestion, absorption, respiration, kidney function, and metabolism are almost entirely new.... Without the kind co-operation of so many friends, it would have been impossible for me to have brought out such a complete revision of the book within the short space of time that has elapsed since the last edition was published. In spite of the introduction of so much new material, the bulk of the volume has not been materially increased, extensive excisions of what has now become antiquated having also been carried out. In bringing the book up to date, I have endeavored to remember that the main object of the work is to supply students with the elementary textbook, although at the same time my aim has been to make it as complete as possible."

The reader will note that when all the chapters on functions listed (and these include ALL the VITAL functions of the body) are almost entirely rewritten, then the reason must have been that there were so many wrong things taught in such chapters previously that it was impossible to merely make corrections. This Twenty-First Edition was published before the World War, since which all physiologies were again completely revised due to the additional knowledge gained at that time that had to replace previously erroneous ideas.

It was only a few years ago, relatively speaking, since forty-eight was the total number of chemical elements; since the atom was accepted as the last division of matter, the indestructible unit, and as the unit upon which all chemistry was based and around which it was organized. Valence, or the attractive power of the atom, was its most peculiar, permanent, and recognizable property, and at that time physiology was in harmony with chemistry. Today, we know that the electron, proton, fields of force, must all be comprehended before we can understand the colloid; that no physiology can even approach correctness until we understand colloids, as we are almost nothing else, and colloid chemistry is a new subject. Its developers are the first to admit that the present-day knowledge of these substances is incomplete, inexact, and subject to radical changes. How then can we expect physiology, which deals with the normal functions of groups of colloids, to be dependable? Great advances have been made, and it is today in line with what we know today – that is the best that can be said of it.

If we cannot understand what the normal function of the body is, if we do not know just what keeps us alive, how then are we going to detect slight variations or correct gross abnormalities? The schools of treatment, medical or nonmedical, are up against this problem. In this teaching we are *not*, because we *permit* the body itself to bring its own healing powers into activity and do nothing else. So long as abnormal conditions exist within the body, just so long will they be discoverable by the methods we lay down, and as our methods certainly and surely make the exact correction most necessary at the moment, we are relieved of the necessity of making any diagnosis whatever, except as it becomes desirable to watch the improvement by means of those well-known indications classified under the general term of diagnosis.

Second – Diagnosis is difficult because it must always depend to some extent upon the statements the patient or someone familiar with the facts will make, and for numerous reasons these statements are not always reliable, frequently meant to conceal, and almost uniformly directed at the trouble the patient is most concerned about at the moment and not at the underlying trouble. In addition to all of this, the medical doctor is in difficulty in selecting treatment because his remedies are colloidal in nature and have their effects upon colloids (the body being largely colloidal), and since colloid chemistry is only in a formative development, the action of his remedies must remain in doubt until the particular patient shows his good or bad response or lack of any. How different and more to be desired the instant change that is experienced under the work we teach herein.

To show how exact is the above, we quote from Dr. John V. Shoemaker, author of *Materia Medica and Therapeutics*, professor of Materia Medica, etc., in the Medico-Chirugical College and Hospital of Philadelphia. He says, "Rational Medicine ... is enlightened empiricism," which means that, because a certain drug was found effective in certain dosage and combination in a certain disease and patient, it was accepted as a good drug for that disease – empiricism. The study of that drug so as to observe the effect of its active principle on the tissues involved in that disease led to a certain faint understanding as to why the drug did the things observed – enlightened empiricism.

He goes on to state, "Rational Medicine ... is an enlightened empiricism which is not based on fixed law, but is progressively improving in proportion with advances in other departments of science. Any practice of medicine assuming to rest upon a foundation less broad than this or on a system which is fixed and stationary, by its own terms, separates itself from scientific medicine and makes its followers a medical sect or 'school.' In the course of centuries, many such schools have been brought to light and after a brief period have been outgrown and forgotten. Such a fate is the natural destiny of any restricted system based upon dogma.... Scientific or regular medicine is quite distinct from any school or sect in medicine."

Nevertheless, so-called "Scientific Medicine" is itself only a "school" of the same class and sort as the others the doctor refers to, despite his denial.

Therefore, as Dr. Shoemaker states, Modern Medicine has no fixed principle or basis whatsoever upon which to establish any of its conclusions. It just "growed up" like Topsy. And so we sum up medicine in this brief indication of the material to be found in this chapter by repeating that diagnosis is approximately 50% correct; that diagnosis must be 100% correct before any hope of correct treatment can be held; and that correct treatment is based upon "enlightened empiricism" without the slightest "dogma," that is, without the slightest conception as to what it is all about.

No wonder that everyone who consistently relies upon medical care exclusively is finally *forced* by constantly increasing dis-ease to abandon it in favor of one of the drugless methods, the operating table, or the graveyard, and this last alternative, they arrive much before the time they should, even accepting for the sake of argument the three score and ten years the Bible allots.

The medical doctor recognizes his limitations but is very slow to admit it, but Jerome Alexander, M. Sc., Consulting Chemist and Chemical Engineer; Past Chairman, Committee of the Chemistry of Colloids; Fellow of the American Institute of Chemists; Member of the American Institute of Chemical Engineers; American Institute of Mining and Metallurgical Engineers, etc., states in his book *Colloid Chemistry* in 1929 under Chemo-Therapy, "We will never trace their effects on the body colloids – a most formidable task. Many remedies operative in vivo do not work in vitro.

"All diseases are caused by, or involve, changes in the body colloids which, though delayed by the presence of protective substances, are sometimes irreversible. To cure the disease, we must remove the cause and aid the tissues and body fluids or 'humors,' as they used to be called, to return to their normal state of dispersion and swelling. Bacteria and other invading organisms, as well as the body tissues, have highly specific adsorptive powers and the 'shot-gun' method of try, miss and try again is our main reliance in finding something that will kill the germ or disease and spare the patient."

He also quotes Sir William Bateson in his address before the British Association for the Advancement of Science as saying, "Every theory of evolution must be such as to accord with the facts of physics and chemistry, a primary necessity to which our predecessors paid small heed.... Of the physics and chemistry of life we know next to nothing. Somehow the characters of living things are bound up in properties of colloids and are largely determined by the chemical powers of enzymes, but the study of these classes of matter has only just begun. Living things are found by simple experiment to have powers undreamt of, and who knows what may be behind?"

Osteopathy was based upon the conception that congestion was the cause of disease. Dr. A.T. Still, the founder of osteopathy said, "The blood is the life;" "The reign of the artery is supreme;" and osteopathy really embraced the FIRST DEFINITE IDEA, expressed the first definite conception of, and provided the first definite method for the CORRECTION of DISEASE as distinguished from its TREATMENT.

It is now known that the "congestion" of the osteopath actually exists, that such areas are more highly acid than they should be or than the immediately adjacent areas; that the capillaries within such areas are closed and remain closed longer than they should; that the mechanism which alternately opens and closes them is "out of gear" due to this acid accumulation; and that in fact the old-fashioned, once practiced, but now generally abandoned osteopathic manipulations undoubtedly did move the congested blood and thereby rest and restore the alkalinity of such areas.

Chiropractic was next, with a broad conception. Dr. D.D. Palmer, the discoverer of this work, said concerning it that slightly slipped vertebrae in the human spine produced pressures on nerves emitting from the spinal column on their way from the brain to the tissue cell, thereby shutting off the life forces necessary to the cell to maintain function and that all disease and the symptoms thereof, including the "congestion" of the osteopath, were traceable to this cause.

It is now known that the loss of "Mental Impulse" in the tissue cell, which Dr. Palmer ascribed to the pressure of a bone on the nerve carrying such impulse, DOES NOT OCCUR.

It is known that the nerve does not come under any considerable compression by any slight slipping of any vertebra on account of the bedding of all such nerves in a protective fatty covering as they emit from the spine and on their passage through the opening. It is also known that the idea Dr. Palmer proposed that the brain converted "life forces" from the universal forces and supplied each tissue of the body with this force and that this supply was the total supply that any tissue could have so that any interference with that supply meant disease and lack of function at the place in proportion where and as the nerve carrying it normally ended IS ALL ERRONEOUS because the nerve itself as a transmission line is incapable of transmitting any such great amounts of force. It DOES transmit small electrical impulses amounting to 5 to 50-millionths of a volt, according to Dr. Detler W. Bronk of the University of Pennsylvania, that set in motion the power machinery of the cell, tissue, or organ, and without the activating impulse there is no response.

The typical response, however, may be elicited by means of very small electric impulses or by any means of stimulation other than electrical, through the nerve, through adjacent tissues, or if directly applied to the tissue itself, as any well-conducted experiment will invariably demonstrate, thus proving erroneous the idea that the evanescent, intangible, almost spiritual thing that Palmer talks about is totally imaginary and is not in any sense the thing it is said to be.

This does not mean to say that there is no such Universal Force or even that the human brain or body is unadapted or incapable of making such a contact as Palmer suggests. But it is a purely speculative and philosophical idea that has absolutely no importance in health or disease at the present time, for it has been amply demonstrated that independent tissues, both in or out of the human body and not connected with any transforming unit such as Palmer imagines the brain to be, continues to live and thrive just as though they were so connected, an activity which would be totally impossible if Palmer's theory were correct.

Amongst those who have experienced the wonderful results sometimes accomplished by the chiropractor, there will be many who will question these statements because how then could the chiropractor get the results he does?

This very question was the one that led to the correct answer, which is that in his attempt to move a vertebra which was slightly out of place, being held there by an abnormal muscular pull, the drive concentrated upon that vertebra is transmitted through that muscle and the fundamental correction of the sacrum is accidentally and automatically made. This occurs in the successful cases but frequently fails to occur. This is the reason why of two identical cases under the same chiropractor at the same time, each receiving his best care, one makes a startling recovery and the other fails to improve. If it happened that the chiropractor "adjusted" the right vertebra in exactly the right direction, the additional tension instantly thrown upon the already overstrained muscle which was pulling that vertebra out of its normal position was frequently great enough to cause the necessary correction of the sacrum in at least that one direction, the vertebra remained "adjusted," the patient recovered from that complaint, and everyone concerned believed that it was the movement of the vertebra that produced the result, because the movement of the sacrum, being painless, easy, and noiseless, was completely overshadowed by the directly opposite sense of the vertebra. It might be interesting to some to know that this slipping of the sacrum occurred more frequently under the heavy adjusting on the two-piece table of a few years ago and explains the reason why there are fewer startling cures made at the present time amongst those using chiropractic or similar methods.

Our idea is that this overstretched muscle is also responsible for the "acid areas" which exist around the congestion of the osteopath. Jerome Alexander states, "If anything prevents the capillary from opening again at the proper time, we have a vicious circle – an 'acid' capillary surrounded by 'acid' tissue – leading to congestion or inflammation." But the osteopath of today, having absorbed the teaching of the chiropractors and all other manipulative methods and having made these teachings part of their own books, have finally abandoned all of it and have become osteopathic physicians and surgeons, which means that they have discarded the conceptions that gave osteopathy its claim to separate method and now favor the "enlightened empiricism" of the medical profession.

The medical people have recognized for many years past – and are recognizing more and more – the fact that distortion or lack of symmetry of the body plays an important part in disease because definite types of distortion are always present in each and every disease. But their training is not sufficient along mechanical lines to allow the rapid and intelligent development of this idea. The osteopaths began and the chiropractors have continued along these lines but never developed it to its logical conclusion.

It took the combined experiences of the osteopaths, coupled with Dr. Hurley's in wide and varied experience and knowledge as an engineer as well as seventeen years of continuous practice as a chiropractor, to allow rapid development along these mechanical lines. We have only begun, but this present work is far in advance of anything known before, as you will readily appreciate when you develop the understanding and skill required to practice this method.

No one can afford to be ignorant of the facts contained in this book. Our aim is to teach you to measure and understand the presence of weaknesses in the human body that predispose to illnesses of all kinds. By seeing them and measuring them in advance, we teach you to correct them before serious troubles develop. If the troubles have already developed, the method is still equally effective in restoring the body to normal. This is truly preventive.

CHAPTER II...FACTS AND CONCEPTS[2]

The sun and all the worlds, the rocks, the ocean, and man are all made of matter. Only the rate of vibration and the forms change. This change in the highest development known to us results in man. Without matter in a high state of development, there is no consciousness and without consciousness, there is no pain, no dis-ease.

All matter is subject to fatigue. When fatigue increases to the point of exhaustion, the thing that was ceases to be. Worlds and all they contain disappear. Bridges, buildings, ships and automobiles go on the scrap pile, and men go to the graveyard.

When normal loads are imposed upon any structure, that is, loads that fall within the "elastic limit" of the structure, only stresses are set up within that structure and it is said to be in a state of *stress* from which no distortion results. But if such loads are increased, whether gradually or suddenly, beyond the "elastic limit" of the structure, *strains* are set up and the structure is immediately deflected beyond its ability to restore itself to normal. It is then said to be *strained* and is then *permanently distorted*, due to cellular and intercellular changes (strains) that have occurred.

---

[2] Many concepts in this and subsequent chapters were later given specific definitions by Dr. Hurley. See Glossary.

Unless definite and appropriate means for removing these strains are adopted, it will make no difference whether the abnormal load is removed immediately or permitted to remain; exhaustion and complete destruction will occur. The distortions above referred to are permanent and the structure has undergone degenerative changes, which ultimately by exhaustion will destroy it. It may not fall down at once of its own weight if the abnormal loads are *immediately* removed, but unless the distortion is corrected, its *usefulness* is over. This is true of ALL MATTER, and these changes in men lead to DEATH.

In man, performance of work or any of the activities of life within the "elastic limit" of the individual concerned leads only to further development and greater strength, but as soon as the load is increased beyond that limit, whether by a slowly increasing load of work, worry, or care, or suddenly by violence from falls, blows, breaks, or strains, distortion occurs. The body that suffers it becomes disabled exactly as the bridge or building does and the same reason for the distortion exists, viz: CELLULAR and INTERCELLULAR STRAIN. This disability, which may take the form of any acute or chronic disease, temporary, periodical, or permanent, all indicating some degree of exhaustion and some degree of disability exactly proportionate to the degree of distortion, must exist. Not all distortions of the human body are apparent to the untrained observer, and people who are sick may be and frequently are certain that they are not thus distorted. But later in this volume we will show how to determine the fact, so that even the previously untrained may not only see but also analyze and correct.

Also, there are many distortions so great as to show a true deformity and yet the individual may be able to get about and perform certain amounts and kinds of work, apparently as free from disease and distress as the average person, and the question may arise how this can be. The answer is that such people *never* have the abilities their own bodies would manifest if not so deformed; that they are more subject to disease than they would be if not so deformed; that they are always fatigued when they should be rested; and finally, that if the condition has begun during formative years, a very great deal of compensation has been made to their advantage. This subject will be again referred to in our present work.

Most of these distortions have passed unnoticed until now because this volume, for the first time in the history of the healing art, systematizes the investigation of them and shows in detail the manner of their correction and bases a complete system for the restoration of health upon their observation and correction. Naturally, small attention was paid to matters for which no correction was known. They became simply a part of the unavoidable difficulties of life, but now that the correction is possible, certain and easy, it is quite important to look about you and see that hardly any person is free from some degree of distortion, regardless of age or condition, and this is the true reason why no one is well.

Man has always known that distortion signified dis-ease probably because a broken bone or a strained joint was painful and because as soon as pain disappeared he was again able to assume his upright posture. Hence, pain and dis-ease have occupied his attention since the earliest times.

All distortions of the human body can be observed in many ways and at many points. One of the conditions where distortion is easy to see is in the spine where such troubles produce curvature, and very frequently slight curvatures are called "occupational curvatures." In reality there is no such thing. Our experience is now so extensive that we are able to make that statement with authority. Every such condition will disappear without any change of habit or employment under the methods herein completely explained and taught, and every diseased condition present in the body will disappear in exact proportion as this is accomplished.

Due to entirely new concepts as to the effects of these distortions on the body, we now understand them as the *causative factors* in functional and organic disease. As long ago as 1810, Samuel Hahnemann, the great founder of homeopathy, said in his *Organon of the Rational Art of Healing*:

"The physician has no higher aim than to make sick folk well, to pursue what is called the Art of Healing.

"The highest ideal of cure is the speedy, gentle and enduring restoration of health, or the removal and annihilation of disease in its entirety, by the quickest, most trustworthy and least harmful way, according to principles that can readily be understood (the rational art of healing).

"He is also a maintainer of health, if he knows the causes that may disturb health and excite disease and how to remove them from healthy persons.

"It may be granted that every disease must depend upon an alteration in the inner working of the human organism. This disease can only be mentally conceived through its outward signs and all that these signs reveal; in no way whatever can the disease itself be recognized.

"The invisible disease producing alteration in the outward man, together with the visible alteration in health (the sum of symptoms), make up that which is called disease; both together actually constitute the disease.

"The invisible disease-producing change in the inward man and the complex of outwardly perceptible symptoms are consequently determined by one another reciprocally and inevitably; both together make up the disease in its entirety, that is, constitute such a unity that the latter must stand or fall simultaneously with the former, that they must exist together and disappear together, so that whatsoever is able to call out a group of definite symptoms must have caused in the body that corresponding inward morbid change which is inseparable from the outward appearance of disease. Otherwise the appearance of the symptoms would be impossible; and similarly whatever removes permanently the complex of outward signs of disease, must simultaneously have removed the inward morbid change, because the banishing of the former without the disappearance of the latter is inconceivable."

These distortions are the unfailing indices that Dr. Hahnemann sensed but never found. The distortions and their correction, which this volume teaches, continued to engage the minds of men, and in 1874 Dr. A.T. Still announced the school of osteopathy. He taught the recognition of some distortions and means for partially correcting some of them. Unfortunately, his successors, finding conditions they could not identify or correct, have taken the wrong road and, instead of discovering just where their troubles lay, have adopted all sorts of auxiliary methods to improve results, finally losing sight almost entirely of their original principles. The chiropractors have done exactly the same thing, and this book again brings the subject back to its broad fundamentals, and shows how to do the thing all others have tried and failed to do.

For some years, Dr. Henry P. de Forest of New York City, and Dr. Horace G. Baldwin of Tannersville, NY, have been conducting researches in the medical laboratories of Cornell University to develop the consistency with which results can be obtained by adjustment of the sacrum, having noted the frequently startling effects of the correct adjustment of this bone by osteopaths and chiropractors. They have, during this time, observed and cared for considerably over 3000 selected cases. Their results have been reported to have been entirely satisfactory in practically every case. They are hunting for the anatomical explanation, basing their search on the chiropractic idea of nerve pressures. The true explanation of these cures is cellular and intercellular strain, and when that fact is recognized and corrective technic rendered exact, as herein taught, results will be exactly uniform in every case.

Now let us go on with our strains. Metals distorted by strain and near their breaking point, that is, fatigued nearly to the point of exhaustion, can be restored to full usefulness again, and so can men. In both cases the process is identical and consists in first removing the abnormal load, and then correcting the abnormal cellular and intercellular tensions produced therein by these abnormal loads and evidenced by the distortions. In metals, this is done by heat. In men, by rest. In both cases the correction demands intelligent application. Just throwing a cutting tool into an oil bath after having heated it is no heat treatment and will not restore the tool. Just doping a man to sleep in spite of pain and giving him a colonic irrigation or sweat bath will not rest or "rest-ore" the man.

The cellular and intercellular tensions must be corrected so as to remove all strain, destroy all distortion, correct all disabilities, rehabilitate all vital powers, in short, bring all matter – ships, buildings, or men – back to maximum usefulness in exact proportion as it is accomplished, by the correction of FATIGUE.

Cellular and intercellular stress is normal and necessary. It is these stresses that by cohesion produce form, texture, and quality, and support function. Cellular and intercellular *strain* is abnormal and destructive. It is these strains that by crystallization produce deformity, change texture, and destroy quality and function in metals and in men. In living tissues, this crystallization takes on the characteristics of decay and this decay is known as organic disease.

Thus in functional disease, this crystallization or decay is in its incipient form; and rest only is necessary for its correction. When, however, this same process is allowed to continue until the decay itself is important, then the condition has reached the point where it is known as organic disease, and *rest plus reconstruction* is necessary.

But ships and buildings are made of matter which is without power of growth and the resulting and co-related ability to repair itself, and it is here that living tissue becomes superior for it has this ability, and fatigue does not reach the stage of exhaustion except through extreme and immediate violence, until the organism becomes poisoned by its own wastes. This poisoning is unnecessary, abnormal, and wrong. Among animals, man has the superior intelligence, and when he becomes sufficiently intelligent he will no longer permit this abnormality and may even develop IMMORTALITY.

In all matter, stresses are normal, strains abnormal. Stresses do not destroy because they do not distort. The opposite is true of strains, and hence we develop these concepts:

Exhaustion is the only cause of Death.

Degrees and amounts of Fatigue measure the approach of Exhaustion.

Fatigue is some degree of Exhaustion.

Disease is some degree of Death.

Degrees and amounts of disease measure the approach of Death.

Fatigue and Disease are here synonymous.

Let us call attention to the effect of weariness upon posture, to the parallel between the bent, twisted, distorted bodies that weariness produces, and the bodies of aged, elderly and sick people, that is, those nearly exhausted and nearing death. The sure measure of the approach of death is the measure of effectiveness. A man's energy, vitality, ability, and effectiveness are very clearly measured for all to see in his posture, his mode and relative speed of action, and the coordination or lack of it that he shows. This is true because man is an upright animal and any departure from erectness indicates by its degree and permanence the amount of fatigue his body has accumulated. When it is increased to the point where movement is entirely impossible, he borders upon exhaustion, and this is known to all as the proof of imminent death.

A striking example is brought to our attention by John Hix in *Strange as it Seems* when he tells of a Thomas Hall of

Cambridge, England, born in 1741 and died of old age September 1747. "His appearance was like that of an old man, his head being completely bald and his face full of wrinkles.

"The following inscription, in Latin, was placed on his tombstone: 'Stop, traveler, and wondering, know here buried lie the remains of Thomas, the son of Thomas and Margaret Hall: who not one year old had signs of manhood; not three and was almost four feet high; endued with uncommon strength, a just proportion of parts and a stupendous voice; before six died as it were of advanced age.'"

Man's posture and effectiveness are more truly a measure of age than is the number of years that have passed over his head. Some people are old at 30 and a few are young at 60, in both mind and body. Age is accumulated weariness – fatigue.

You wake up in the morning feeling as well as usual and continue to until you stoop to pick up a shoe, when something lets go. You are immediately suffering pain in the back, and depending upon its location, you are said to have an attack of lumbago, sciatica, neuritis, stiff neck, etc. Frequently this is so severe that you cannot move at all for some time, and if it is not improved, you are likely to have real trouble with it, because it prevents rest.

In these cases, the body immediately loses its upright posture and becomes more or less distorted. In some mild cases, rest alone produces restoration. In others that are more severe, active methods must be added, because the slip that was felt, increased to a serious degree, a distortion already existing and the condition now is such that, even if it passes off without special effort on your part, it will leave plenty of trouble behind it with a noticeable degree of distortion, thus actually taking years of life out of your body.

Hold out your arm and notice how short a time elapses before pain begins. Is this a "congested area?" Is it a "pinched nerve?" Should a pain tablet or hypodermic be used? Should an operation be performed? Or should you put the arm at rest?

When drowning, fatigue rapidly increases because the lungs are becoming filled with water, thus reducing the oxidizing power of the body, until the slightest motion is so painful as to make effort almost impossible. Death by drowning is by no means the easy death so many people believe it to be. But in such cases where death does not result, no serious distortion occurs, and hence recovery is rapid and usually very complete, for rest is possible, and this is the essential difference between this condition and the case of the man who gets a "kink in his back." This man has sustained distortions and cannot rest, and if no correction is made, he is certain to have repeated attacks, each one leaving added distortion. Soon, although only forty, he will walk like a man of sixty or eighty and look and feel of like age. He will actually be eighty in effectiveness.

Consider two prize-fighters. They go into the ring in the best physical condition it is possible for them to attain. If no lucky blow is struck and the fight progresses normally, it is only a few rounds until you see both fighters lose some of their elasticity, speed and coordination, and when near the end of a hard battle, both bodies are suffering pain due to the fatigue sustained and neither is able to hit with even a small part of the force that was at his command when he began, or with the same accuracy. If one of them is able to gather himself up and deliver just one blow with anything like his original power and accuracy, it is a "knock-out," though his opponent absorbed many such blows at the beginning without any particular distress.

In all these cases, it is apparent that falls, blows or labor which would have no apparent effect upon a man of good condition would entirely destroy life if sustained at the moment of gravest fatigue, that is, the moment when the ability to maintain the upright posture was at its lowest ebb, when the distortion was greatest, and so we come to realize that "Degrees and amounts of Fatigue measure the approach of Exhaustion," and that "Fatigue is some degree of Exhaustion."

We have excepted lethal injuries from this discussion, but such injuries produce the same result by causing large electrical changes and vital losses, and some diseases cause almost equally rapid vital losses – as cholera – all resulting in exhaustion.

Any condition that robs the body of its water or interferes with the flow of fluids of the body, whether it results in a collection or in a drying-out of certain areas, is a dangerous source for the accumulation of fatigue and may become an immediate cause of exhaustion. The danger from the loss of blood arises from these principle factors. (1) Loss of fluid; (2) Acidosis – due to loss of red corpuscles with their oxidizing property; (3) Loss of protection against infective processes due to loss of white corpuscles; (4) Reduction of electrical negativity and ionizing power; (5) Loss of alkaline reserve.

Energy is restored to bodies almost completely exhausted from injury or shock by the replacement of the fluid of the body by the injection of a normal salt solution into the veins. Because the normal spleen in a normal body will produce not less than 2,000,000 red corpuscles per hour for a short period of time in any case when the air becomes less dense, as ascending in an airplane, this loss is soon repaired. White corpuscles are in such superabundance at all times that if the exhaustion is taken care of by methods already indicated, no danger need be feared from loss of immunity to infection.

Fatigue and disease are here synonymous and so we list opposite each other the signs of fatigue and disease that everyone knows:

Mild Fatigue	Signs	Mild Disease
Yes	Prostration	Yes
Yes	Rapid Pulse	Yes
Yes	Thirst	Yes
Yes	Loss of appetite	Yes
Yes	Dull mentality	Yes
Yes	Supersensitive	Yes
Yes	Poor Bowel Action	Yes
Yes	Dry skin	Yes
Yes	Some pain	Yes

As fatigue or disease increases, these signs are intensified and the dis-ease is felt chiefly in the part of the body most fatigued, and so takes on different characteristics as it progresses because of the peculiar functions of the different parts of the body interfered with. For instance, influenza. The first sign of importance in the diagnosis of this disease is a degree of prostration (fatigue) out of all proportion to the apparent gravity of the trouble. The only loss of function that occurs early is poor bowel action. But as the dis-ease (that is, the fatigue) continues to progress, the intestinal symptoms become predominant in some cases, liver in others, lung in another, bronchial, nasal, mental, etc. In each person the disease shows its main symptoms, its greatest damage, and its greatest prostration in the area of greatest fatigue, and the signs of fatigue are embraced in the evidences of disease until exhaustion (death) occurs or recuperation begins, when again the fatigue is the only remaining sign as it was the first sign of oncoming trouble.

Now the indirect evidence. If exhaustion is the only cause of death, then it must be true that without exhaustion there would be no death; without fatigue, no exhaustion, no disease, and consequently not even an approach to death. That is, man would live as long as he was able to maintain this ideal state or until some accident inflicted sufficient injury to immediately kill him – again by exhaustion.

For more than nineteen years (since 1912) the Rockefeller Institute has been conducting an experiment in which chicken hearts, livers, kidneys, skin, etc., have been kept alive and functioning on glass slides, totally disconnected from any living organism. These tissues not only continue to live, but carry on all the processes for which they were needed in the chicken's body. They have already lived far beyond the time when any chicken possessing them would have died, and they have grown at such a rate that the new tissue must constantly be cut away and destroyed to prevent the specimen from becoming unwieldy – for in the case of the chicken heart, it doubles its size every forty-eight hours when kept under ideal conditions.

More, there is no sign of any aging and it appears that there is no reason to expect any such development. More important still, it has been proven that such tissue will gradually grow back to normal even if it was diseased when the experiment began, and the only care these tissues require is that a constant temperature favorable to them shall be maintained; that they shall be washed with various fluids to furnish them the food elements they require; to clean them of their own poisonous waste products; and to provide the proper rest. The same experiment has been carried out so many times and by so many operators and always with the same result that the opinion of the scientist that the cell is immortal seems dependable and justified. If the human cell is immortal, then the human body has all the machinery at hand and the intelligence to properly control it to maintain these ideal conditions. There seems to be no reason why it should not operate as efficiently so long as the four essentials above noted are satisfactorily supplied. However, lacking any one of the four, fatigue begins. Fatigue continuing, disease becomes apparent. And still continuing, exhaustion, which is death, rapidly follows.

The proposition that disease is some degree of death is so familiar to everyone that small argument is necessary. "I'm dead tired," is the literal truth. And so we feel that we have established our concept that "Fatigue and Disease are here synonymous."

It is necessary to form a very clear understanding of these concepts because this whole method is not in any sense chiropractic or osteopathy, or any one of the older healing arts. It is a totally new system, based upon these concepts and unless they are completely and thoroughly understood, your practical application of the technic will be faulty. In exact proportion as that fault exists, results will fail to be obtained and even damage may occur, for this work is very potent. You will see case after case report instant and immediate changes, and they are always to some degree permanent. That potential exists, and it depends considerably upon your knowledge and acceptance of these concepts whether it will be potential for good or bad.

CHAPTER III...CONTINUATION OF CONCEPTS

Excepting direct nerve injury,
Pain is the earliest symptom of Disease.
Fatigue is the only cause of Pain.
Pain has no other origin than muscular tissue.
Muscular tissue is the origin of Disease.

We except direct nerve injury because in the normal body no nerve can be directly injured, exactly as no blood vessel can be directly injured, since to reach a nerve or vessel it is necessary to bruise or break the covering structures. Nerve exhaustion does not occur and nervous diseases will be separately discussed.

It is frequently said that a certain man suffered a "nervous breakdown." There is no such thing. Every time a disability is so diagnosed, it is an admission that the diagnostician does not know what is wrong with the patient. This is true of Neurasthenia, and, when anyone is treated for such a condition, he may be sure he will not get well, because the disease is a mystery to the one in whom he puts his faith. Remember it is a physiological fact that there is no such disease and no such condition as "Nervous Exhaustion." Even in true death by starvation, the nervous system loses only 3% of its bulk and instead of becoming less active and able, becomes more so. The will to live manifests thus in a greater ability to secure the means to live. Neurasthenia is only excessive fatigue resulting in hypersensitiveness.

As previously indicated, pain really acquaints a person with the fact that he has disease. It is pain that robs him of his ease. Without the pain he is not conscious of the presence of disease. Lung trouble does not cause pain in the lung unless the pleura, the sack that contains the lung, is involved and becomes inflamed. There is no way for the person to know that his lungs are sick until the disease has already caused considerable damage. The same is true in kidney troubles and in every trouble where the organ involved is poorly supplied with muscular fibers. On the other hand, every organ well supplied with such tissue makes a great fuss and causes plenty of disease as soon as the muscular fibers there are subjected to any strain, exactly as the muscles in your arm begin to hurt as soon as you overtire them.

The brain, the ductless glands, the spleen, and the liver are the other organs poorly supplied with muscular tissue and these organs never hurt. They may produce vague feelings of weight or distress due to encroachment of or upon surrounding muscular tissue, but they never set up the fierce agonizing pains that all the other parts of the body are subject to. Headaches are not pains in the brain. A very large tumor may exist in the brain itself without causing any severe pain. The skull may be depressed by fracture, but it is not the pressure *on the brain* that hurts so terribly. It is the condition in which this misfortune leaves the muscular structures involved by the depression.

Our next concept that fatigue is the only cause of pain is partly the result of observation in the developmental stages of this work and now sufficiently demonstrated to *require* acceptance. We find that pain always arises when muscular structure becomes fatigued. Its intensity is directly proportional to the amount of fatigue sustained and we find that it is controlled or removed in exact proportion as the fatigue is removed. We should understand here that fatigue results from blows and other injuries sustained as easily and surely as it does from excessive or extraordinary use, and in this statement we use the word fatigue in its broadest sense. It here includes all the physiological evidences that we will discuss shortly.

"Pain has no other origin than muscular tissue." Of course, it is well known that "nerve platelets" or "pain corpuscles" set up the vibration which the nerves carry and which is interpreted in the brain as a painful sensation arising at the place where the platelet is. We know that curare, Indian arrow poison, does not destroy this connection though it does destroy the power of motion, and therefore an animal so poisoned cannot move, yet suffers pain as acutely as a normal animal would. We know that opium and anesthetics do destroy this nerve platelet connection and an animal so poisoned feels no pain and makes no movement. We know that there is no other means for setting up the pain vibration than through these platelets or by direct nerve injury. We have made careful search and failed to find these platelets present in any other than muscular tissue. True, we have not found direct evidence that they exist nowhere else, but also we have found no direct evidence that they do exist elsewhere. We have such immediate and positive evidence that any pain can be instantly stopped by causing muscular relaxation as is done in our "contact" that, until certain evidence to the contrary is produced, we believe we are justified in the statement that pain has no other origin than muscular tissue.

Then, too, there are many commonly known facts such as the following:

An ovary or appendix may be chronically diseased, yet cause acute suffering only when some additional stress unusual even to the individual is thrown upon it.

A heart may have leaky valves, yet cause its owner distress and apprehension only at long intervals and under the same conditions.

A muscle in the leg, arm, neck, or back may hurt only at long intervals when the contraction or stress becomes contracture or strain, and under the same conditions as above.

And also, if our concepts are true, then all those organs and parts freely supplied with muscular tissue can and will hurt more frequently and more severely than those parts poorly supplied with muscle, and that is true. In addition, the pain must be proportional to the amount of muscle involved and the degree of involvement, and that also is true. The heart, which is almost entirely muscle and is a most vital organ, gives rise to the most agonizing pain (True Angina Pectoris) that the human body can have. The brain, equally vital but practically devoid of muscular structure, gives rise to no pain at all, and so on.

The character and amount of pain suffered is determined by and proportional to the character of and the amount of the muscular tissue involved. Relief from pain can be secured by massage, hot packs, electro-therapy, medicine, etc. Anything that will produce *relaxation* in the contracted area will give relief from pain and produce rest. Rest is the antidote for fatigue, and when rest progresses to a certain point, "restoration" begins, and the patient recovers.

This work presents a method of securing that relaxation, rest, and rest-oration in every case. It goes further and nearly approaches the ideal because it makes possible the correction that renders the above permanent.

And here we come to the end of the present argument, for the simplest and most self-evident things are the most difficult to prove. And we know that in a strict sense of the word this concept is not conclusively proven – yet there are other significant ideas. For instance, to prove *absolutely* that a straight line is the shortest distance between two points, you must prove that no Infinite Mind may imagine any shorter distance that is beyond the finite mind to grasp, and which, of course, is impossible. Even the two halves of four are not identical. They must be capable of proved equality; otherwise they are not halves. But in *absolute fact* they are not identical and so we "prove" what we argue about or discuss only insofar as we harmoniously correlate it with all other "facts" known to pertain to the subject and already acceptable, and hence we feel that we have reasonably established our concept that:

Pain has no other origin than Muscular Tissue.

So far as direct nerve injury is concerned, such as results from dental work, surgical interference, etc., they all must damage or destroy the integument, and the pain even in these cases may be finally found in muscular tissue. These matters remain for further research.

Now, if muscular tissue is the only source of pain and pain is the earliest symptom of disease, then it necessarily follows that muscular tissue is the origin of disease and that disease has no other origin.

The sacrum has the most powerful muscles of the body attached to it and these muscles are in balance, therefore free from pain, only when the sacrum is exactly in the position normal to it. Any slightest deviation disturbs this balance and puts one or more of these muscles under continuous stretch, which is destructive to it so far as the condition of the muscle from a physiological standpoint is concerned, exactly as continuous contraction without rest does, because such muscles, or a man possessing such muscles, cannot rest. Physiologists state that muscles are highly extensible because of their great ability to restore themselves to normal length and girth after considerable deformation. But muscles are almost completely inextensible as regards their power to grow into or adapt themselves to a greater distance between their bony attachments or their origin and insertion.

It is one of the functions of these muscles to change the relative position of one part of the body to that of some other part. The muscle thus, to use a crude illustration, plays the part of a man on the end of a lever, each joint furnishing the fulcrum around which the lever operates. Just as the man must have some solid point to stand on, a fulcrum around which to exercise his power, and a movable point for the lever to effect; so the muscle must have a part of the body which does not move (point of origin) and a fulcrum (formed by the joint) and some other part of the body which must move in response to the effort (point of insertion). So it will be seen that at least insofar as the skeletal muscles are involved, there is no purpose in attaching both ends of a muscle to the same bone, for if this were done the only effect of contracture, which is the normal activity of muscle, would be merely a bending effect upon that bone. And so we see that the relative position of the bones to which the two ends of a muscle are attached must remain in normal relationship, be restored to such relationships, or reflect their difference in abnormal conditions imposed upon the muscle that attaches to them.

If these two points normally are, say, six inches apart, and some force changes the skeletal relationships to six and a quarter inches, the muscle does not change its length and grow into a normal condition of its minute structure so long as it is forced to bear this stretch. It is difficult to make this point clear, yet the whole of disease and its explanation hinges upon the proper conception of just this idea.

Expressed differently, we might say that when a muscle is at rest in the living body, it is constantly and normally in a state of mild stretch. When it is in action, it is in a state of contraction, being shorter than at first, and then in a state of extension, being longer than at first. When action ceases, it goes back to a state of tonicity and mild stretch. It is only when the tissues are in this condition of mild stretch [tonicity] that the wastes accumulated during action are removed and new tissues built to replace those destroyed by the activity. If a muscle is under a stretch that is greater than it should be in a state of normal tonicity, the muscle is never able to carry on this repair sufficiently or discharge its own wastes. It lacks the power of growing lengthwise to suit the new conditions imposed upon it, for if it did, we would be truly deformed by only a small amount of distortion, so therefore the muscle is constantly subject to fatigue and the continually increasing accumulation of waste products.

This is the best arrangement that could be made, because otherwise all distortion would become permanent and man would soon cease to be an upright animal, whereas now, the vast majority of distortions gradually yield to the constant pull of these over-stretched muscles, which results to some degree in a spontaneous correction. As soon as the favorable moment arrives, "something slips," the distortion is partially corrected and some degree of health returns. But in those cases where the distortion was too severe to be so minimized, the body makes the best possible adaptation to the condition now imposed upon it and so we see the beginning of all curvatures, all rotations, and all losses of symmetry in the spine and elsewhere throughout the body and the beginning of all disease.

The body functions as an organism. All the organs in it must maintain their own proper relations with every other part of it. Therefore when any curvature begins, some organs are crowded, squeezed, distorted, and rendered to some degree unable to carry on as before. It depends entirely upon the character and extent of the slip at the sacrum what distortions occur at other points, their degree, and their effect. The organs of the lower abdomen are the first affected as a rule, and the effect moves through the legs and through the trunk toward the arms and head in accordance as it moves into the hips and into the spine. To understand exactly what takes place, it is necessary to trace the history of all the diseases that have afflicted a person in his whole lifetime and then watch the changes occurring in the spine and hips as the correction of the sacrum progresses. It cannot be told, but you can always see just how each disease was caused, because if your work is exactly as it should be, you will always give exactly the correction the patient needs at the moment you are called upon to give it, and you will see the body go back through all the changes that marked the development of the condition appertaining thereto upon your first inspection.

Snapshots are almost as valuable a record of these changes as X-ray pictures, for in a miraculously short time the evidences of distortion will be seen to improve, sometimes on the first attempted correction, but in every case in direct proportion as the necessary correction is obtained. This improvement will be due to correction and not just a covering up of the distortion, as found under methods of treatment such as exercise or orthopedic measures. Take any patient so "corrected," have him completely *relax* in the standing position and note the loss of symmetry present, which was only covered up by the muscular development. Another valuable record of these changes may be made by an outline drawing of your patient on a wall, made by having him stand there while you trace. Repeat this as the correction progresses.

If all of this is true, the question next in mind will be, "Do muscles change their length to suit the changing requirements of a growing body before adult years are reached and should some correction occur in this process?" The answer is, "Yes, to a considerable degree, just as in formative period deformities." Thus a child "outgrows" the disease. We do know that the muscles indicative of the so-called "outgrown" disease remain under stretch and can always be felt as hard, comparatively inelastic bands if search is made for them; that they occur and persist in children; that growth or change in stature makes only partial correction and difference as to the relative amount of stretch present, therefore correcting only part of the trouble and leaving some distortion; and that the technic taught corrects all of this, so that in children of all ages the material in this work is equally applicable and productive. It is true that in children too young to cooperate in your effort at correction it is harder to obtain results, but here results follow the inflexible rule and are exactly proportionate to the amount of correction actually accomplished. All of this is preliminary to the discussion of our next group of concepts that:

Muscle is fatigued only by contraction without rest (rest-oration).

Fatigue accumulates acids, which normally are removed from muscle in rest periods. Continuous contraction or stretch prevents this process.

Accumulated fatigue poisons result in Acidosis.

Acidosis is thus a measure of Fatigue and Exhaustion, Disease and Death.

This embraces vital as well as skeletal muscles, voluntary as well as involuntary muscles, and the condition is impossible without exactly equivalent distortion.

Rest — true Rest-oration — is the only cure.

"I'm dead tired!" How often have you said it and heard it? True, it is generally accepted as merely an idiom, but we have observed that all of these "sayings" have a grain of pure truth in them.

Why is it more tiring to stand than to walk? Because standing gives no period of relaxation during which the acids can be moved out of the muscles that produce them.

Why does the heart beat and the lungs breathe all your life long without complaint, except in diseased conditions? Because there is a period of relaxation after every period of contraction, during which the acids are removed. And does the disease that sometimes destroys these organs follow the broad general law herein laid down? It does. Disease in these organs is exactly and only FATIGUE; this fatigue results as just explained; lack of relaxation and rest is the result of the condition that causes similar disturbances in skeletal muscles, and this is the result of mal-position of parts of the skeleton and can be traced back to its primary, causative factor and then corrected, and this book teaches how.

If muscle is capable of restoring itself to normal and discharging its wastes only in rest periods, that is, only when it is in a state of tonic contraction, and it is also true that distortions prevent such rest periods by forcing the muscle to remain in a state of stretch, as has just been pointed out, then the statement in our concepts that muscle is fatigued only by work without rest stands acceptable. Our next idea that the process of fatiguing is marked by the accumulation of acids is plain physiology. The view that this source of acid is the beginning, real cause, of acidosis is merely an extension of reasoning, although it is also one of the original ideas we claim as our own, and acidosis as a measure of fatigue and the approach of exhaustion and of disease and approaching death is clearly acceptable.

Such processes occur in vital as well as skeletal muscle; voluntary as well as involuntary muscle and, as we have shown, are impossible without exactly equivalent distortion.

We also state that muscle will always relax, that is, assume a state of rest, if possible, before fatigue becomes dangerous. When this is impossible, pain begins. If rest continues impossible, disease with definite characteristics manifests itself and, rest still continuing impossible, exhaustion and death ensue. As previously stated, this condition of constant stretch or contracture invariably and necessarily results from any loss of symmetry (distortion) in the human body. Such a loss of symmetry throws constant strain with resulting fatigue upon various muscle groups, thus preventing rest and rest-oration.

These losses of symmetry must and do have their origin in slight slippings of the sacrum, or in cases of fractures or complete dislocation; and can occur nowhere else and do not. To restore health, it is necessary to restore the body to symmetry. Nothing else need be done and nothing short of that will have the desired effect.

It is almost undoubtedly the effect of the sitting position to produce some sort of "contact." It may be this, as much as the relief of the legs, that rests one in this position. It may easily be true that, after sitting or lying for some time in one position, the desire to move or change into some new position is because the sacrum has moved very slightly in response to the original position and now needs a slightly different contact in order to continue the correction of whatever distortions are still present. Certainly with the muscle attachments and pulls, the muscle abilities, function, and troubles that we have developed and taught in our theoretical and philosophical teaching, nothing else or less than this would be expected.

We also claim as our own, by right of inception of idea, investigation, research, systematization, trial, development, proof and publication, a new, complete and reliable health method of much greater efficiency stated herein. And it is to throw a new and truer light upon the processes of living, the state of health and all the vital concerns of every human being, to attempt to make possible the eradication of pain and disease from the human race as promised by the Aquarian-Age Prophets of long ago, that this book is written.

It must not be supposed that a complete education can be compressed within the covers of a single book, and no attempt has been made to do so. But if the student will master this work, we believe he will find himself able then to restore normal health to any person who is sick or diseased, provided only that there is sufficient vitality to keep that patient alive for the short time required for the method herein laid down to become effective.

This book teaches no miracles, and in cases where there is a long-standing structural change, degenerative disease, etc., time must be allowed for the body to rebuild itself. However, ANY PAIN can be CONTROLLED by the proper application of the technic. No person can use tissues destroyed by disease nor get function from organs so damaged until new tissues have been grown. Such processes are amazingly rapid, however, once proper correction is secured and during the period above mentioned, increased and increasing ease and function will be experienced from minute to minute in painful conditions or acute cases; and from day to day in the chronic ones. Every disease can be successfully handled by following the instructions herein laid down, with no expense and no additional equipment.

We offer none of the numerous case histories proving all of the above that are available. We could fill books with nothing but that. But we do advise you to read the balance of this with care and understanding, and then try it on someone, and you will, if you are careful, immediately develop your own proofs.

CHAPTER IV...EVIDENCES OF DISTORTION

If distortion is such an important matter as our previous chapters have indicated, then it is evidently necessary to understand, as nearly as possible, just what would be classed as distortion.

First, look at the back of a person as he stands with feet together, eyes closed, and every muscle as relaxed as possible. Now, construct or imagine a vertical line that falls midway between the heels.

1. Note if the head tilts or turns to one side or the other of this vertical line – which establishes normal. The center of the head should be in exact line with the vertical line.
2. Does the middle of the neck lie exactly on this normal vertical line as it should, or does it curve to one side or the other?
3. The center line of the spine should line up with this normal vertical line also.
4. Is one shoulder lower than the other, or drawn more forward? They should be relaxed and level. Also, the shoulder blades should lie flat and smooth on the ribs and should not project from the body in any way.
5. Is one hip higher than the other? They should be level.

6. Does the line formed midway between the buttocks and the line formed midway between the thighs fall exactly on normal vertical line, as it should?

7. Is one buttock swung further towards the front than the other?

8. Are there hollows at the sides of the hips showing heavily contracted muscles? This is very abnormal and shows that great strain is present and that those muscles have no opportunity to relax and are therefore accumulating fatigue.

9. Are both legs symmetrical all the way down, or does one have a different contour, and is the knee joint of one side further forward than the other?

The normal posture, as viewed from behind, should appear as shown in Figure 1-A.

Now look at your patient from the side and compare with what you see in Figure 1-B, which shows the normal, relaxed posture as viewed from the side. When your body is as perfectly lined up as shown in Figures 1-A and 1-B, you will then be in harmony with the force of gravity and no strain results – no muscles are getting tired, the weight of the body (all weight being determined by the effect of gravity on the mass) falls through the bony and ligamentous structures, and the body can rest, even in the standing position.

The degree and amount of deviation from this normal posture as shown, indicates the degree and amount of fatigue your body is sustaining and accumulating – and accumulated weariness is old age.

When a person is unable to stand with his eyes closed without weaving or swaying, then there is more distortion present than his actual posture shows, for he is unable to relax sufficiently for you to see it. If he did actually relax, his structure would be so out of line that the force of gravity would cause him to fall down. Any structure can lean only to a certain point before it becomes overbalanced and falls down, and once it begins to fall, you know how difficult it is to stop it from falling. Also, when a person is unable to relax at all and tells you he has let down as much as possible, and you find his body very tight and rigid, then the same thing applies. His distortion is so great that if he were to relax he would fall down.

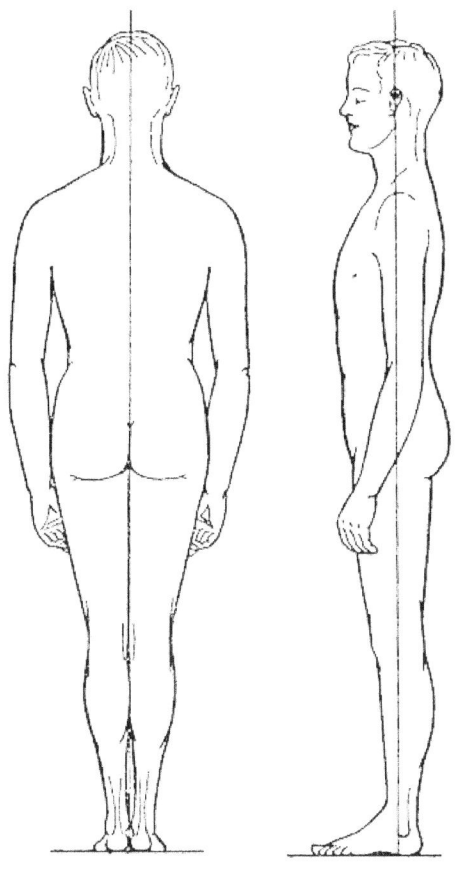

Figure 1-A   *Figure 1-B*

Every distortion present in the body necessitates the *wasting* of the *vital force* in the effort to remain erect, and this destroys the inherent powers of the body by interfering with the normal physiology of muscle. Muscles, as we know them, are really groups of muscular tissue. These groups can be divided again into small bundles; these bundles into the individual muscle cells. These cells are like all cells, characterized by the possession of a cell wall and a body substance known in this case as sarcoplasm.

During activity, parts of the sarcoplasm are changed into sarcolactic acid, which in turn is changed into carbonic acid. If sufficient rest is allowed to that muscle, this carbonic acid is broken up into carbon dioxide and water and discharged from the muscle as rapidly as it is accumulated. As you know, this carbon dioxide is eliminated from the body largely through the lungs. Note the heavy breathing brought on by the presence of fatigue, due either to exercise or distortion.

If the rest is insufficient or the periods too far apart, these acids are incompletely changed and are retained in the muscle because it is only in these rest periods that the necessary change can be made. Acidosis is the term used to describe the condition of the body when such poisons accumulate to the point where their presence is productive of disturbances that are noticeable. Autointoxication is one of the most generally recognized symptoms of acidosis and has erroneously been attributed to constipation and imperfect digestion of food as its major cause, where in truth this is the minor cause, the major one being the retention of the acid waste products in muscles.

Consequently, the proper point of attack for the complete correction of these distortions is of prime importance. It has previously been stated that this point is the *sacrum* and now we must attempt to understand why.

First of all, the sacrum is the structural center of the body. It is around this bone that all of the mechanical movements of the body are centered. From here the weight of the upper part of the body, plus any additional loads carried, is distributed to the legs and transmitted to the ground. It is here that all the movements of any part of the body arise. A known fact to those who have suffered one or more attacks of lumbago is that they quickly discover that the slightest movement of an arm or the head is immediately painful at the junction of the spine and the sacrum. Any load or weight that one picks up in the hands must require more power at this point than at any other because this point must carry the weight of the body, regardless of angle, as well as the additional weight picked up, and this is why, when a man tries to pick up too heavy a load, it is always his "back" that gives out, never his hands or his arms, his feet or his legs, but this point between the spine and the sacrum. This occurs because the body is designed with this slip point to protect other points against breaks.

It is self-evident that if a person was free from distortion, then something would need to slip or break before a distortion of any sort could occur, and if the sacrum represents the "slip point," then it would be reasonable to look to the sacrum for a means of correcting any distortion that had occurred. If, as has been shown, *all pain and disease are the result of distortions*, then a correction of the sacrum, which corrects distortions, would necessarily stop pain and remove the fundamental cause of disease. It is the positive knowledge from practical experience that this occurs that warrants all the preceding.

Let us consider a ship. Figure 2 shows the outline of the hull and the mast stepped in the keelson. Now if the shroud on the right side is too short, then the top of the mast will be pulled to the right, and the mast would appear as the dotted line in Figure 2. Now if a man were put to work who knew nothing about masts and is told to get the top of that mast back in place, he might go to the left shroud and tighten it. This would cause your mast to bend, as shown by the dotted line in Figure 3, and it would likewise spring your keelson and leaks would appear in the hull.

If this mast were to have free movement, it would have to be made in segments, and each segment fastened together and attached and controlled from the deck. This is exactly what we find in the human body. The segments of our spine (mast) are laced together by a muscle called the erector spinae. The spreader in Figure 3 may be likened to our shoulders, which are held in place by the side stay, the latissimus dorsi, which passes from the sacrum to the arm.

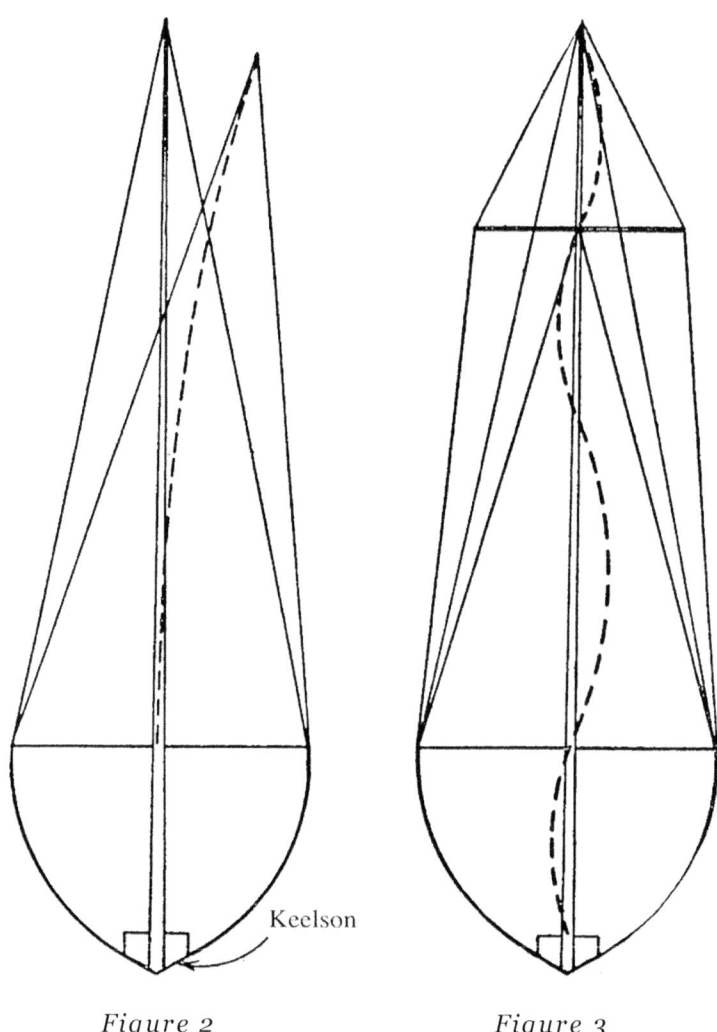

Keelson

Figure 2   *Figure 3*

Now we have something that looks like Figure 4. But suppose we want our boat to go on land. Then we should have to put an apparatus on its sides that would correspond to our hips, and such appendages would certainly be used to further support the mast, and in the body the main muscle that does this is the quadratus lumborum.

We have our back stay (erector spinae) and side stay (latissimus dorsi) and so we must have a front stay, which in the body is supplied by the rectus abdominis, the breast bone, and the sterno-cleido-mastoid muscle. The external and internal oblique muscles as well as the transversalis protect the contents of the abdomen and also help serve as side stays.

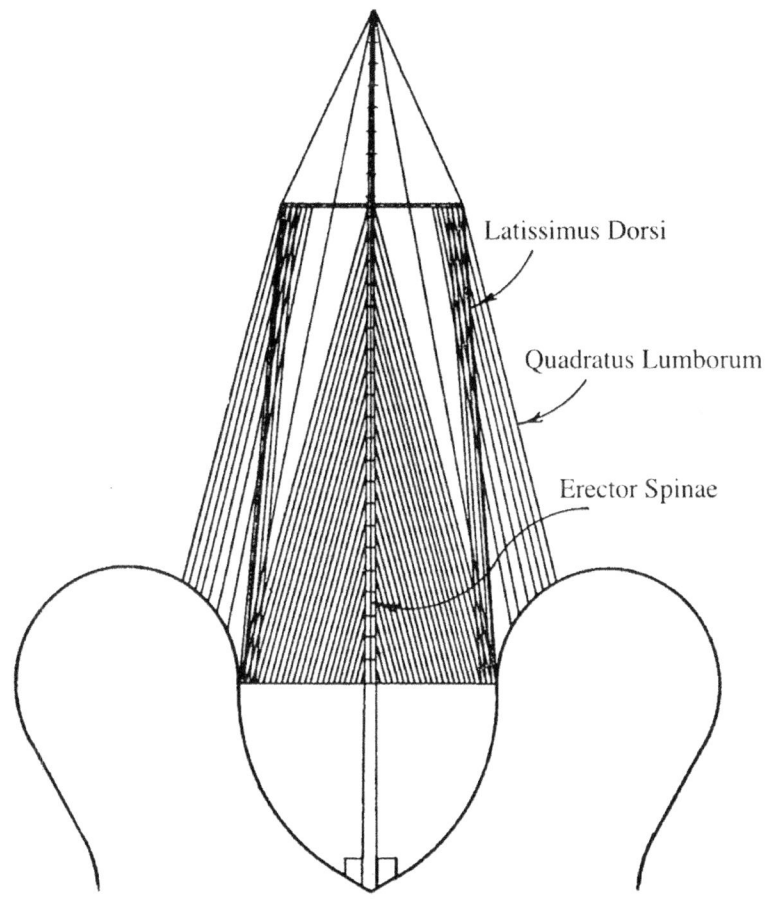

Latissimus Dorsi

Quadratus Lumborum

Erector Spinae

Figure 4

In the body we have the ribs to help brace the structure and to protect the vital organs, and so nature uses them for the attachment of the diaphragm, which forms a big dome and separates the cavity thus formed into two parts, and supports the organs that each part contains. This may be seen in Figure 5.

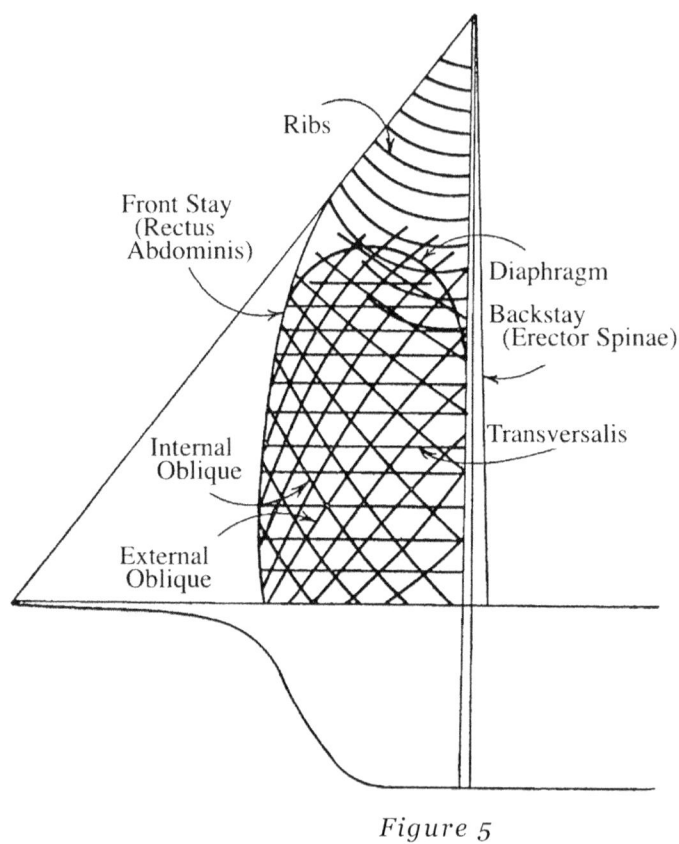

Figure 5

Now it can be readily seen that, if that hull (sacrum) slips downward on the right side between its appendages (hips), immediately the distance between it and the spreader (shoulder), the head, and all the segments (vertebrae) is lengthened so the top of the mast (head) moves to the right side of the body as shown in Figure 2. Now to get the top of the mast back over the hull again, the left stays are tightened, the top of the mast is brought back over the hull, and we have compensated curvature as shown in Figure 3. This also produces a shoving down of the mast, the keelson is sprung and leaks appear in the hull, which are represented by the strained and tender areas found around the sacrum. And this gives a picture of the mechanics of the body.

The spine of man is a flexible and flexuous column, adaptable to all sorts of movement, capable of supporting them and capable, in addition, of supporting and transmitting large additional loads, but it requires balance. Without balance a man, as is common knowledge, loses a large part of his power, and in order to remain in balance, all the muscles that fasten to the base must hold each part of the spine, every vertebra in the spine, with just the right amount of pull.

It has been stated as an anatomical fact that eight muscles fasten to the sacrum, connecting it with all other parts of the body and that all these muscles must remain in exact balance. It has been stated that a muscle lacks the power to grow lengthwise to adapt itself to greater bony distances between its attachment and insertion. It has been shown that, failing to bring these two points into proper relations with each other, they will shift their excess loads to other less resistant muscles and force the body to distribute, as widely as possible, any such excess loads in order to restore to the body some degree of comfort. Otherwise, there would be no recovery from lumbago, except by spontaneous or accidental correction of the trouble. This distribution [adaptation], shifting of trouble from its focal point to distant areas, also permits some rest so not all parts of the body are equally fatigued by any activity. The result is that when a sacrum slips, say toward the feet on the right side of the base, the man will first carry his shoulders and whole upper part of his body to the right of its proper line, but just as soon as this distortion occurs he will bring his body back to a general perpendicular as nearly as possible, by putting some degree of curvature in the lumbar vertebrae, because he must carry his center of weight over his center of force to keep him from falling down. This will be further distributed by the appearance of a secondary curvature in the dorsal and possibly a third one in the cervical region. Each of these curvatures relieves the body and some certain groups of muscles in it of a share of their overburden and imposes some degree of overload on others not previously affected.

The reverse of the above is also true. A severe blow in the shoulder, for instance, may increase an already existing distortion (in which case the body is out of balance) because muscle reacts to any sufficient stimulus by contracting, and blows are mechanical stimuli. Put such stimuli from a sufficiently heavy blow into a muscle already under abnormal conditions and instead of being cushioned by the normal elasticity of muscle, it will be transmitted, exactly as it would be by a steel cable, directly back to the sacrum and there increase the original trouble that had left the muscle in an over-taut or contracted condition. The same thing can happen from an injury to a toe or finger, or any part of the body, or may arise from any vital organ or even strong emotions, such as worry. This is why any slight correction of the sacrum has instant and widespread effect.

The question is often asked, "Why does the light contact make such a great change?" – the word contact being used as is explained in the section on Technic. To understand the answer it is necessary to realize fully all the following:

The body is mostly water. The tissues of the body in a totally relaxed condition are as "trembly" as a dish of gelatin. The proper contact produces, advances, and maintains this relaxation, and it is upon this sort of a mass that the sacrum rests. This alone will show why a very light "contact" will influence it to move slightly in a given direction.

But there is another factor of importance. We have shown that the sacrum cannot move in any degree or direction out of its normal relationships without at the same time throwing one or more of the eight muscles attached to it out of balance and through them other muscles of the body, *all of which are trying their best to correct the faulty condition.* The whole effort of the body is therefore helping to move the sacrum, and when the contact is taken at the right spot and pressed ever so slightly in the right direction, it adds the little additional force required to cause some movement.

There is still another factor. While it is true the sacrum rests on a jelly-like mass and that these muscles are all trying to restore themselves to equilibrium by restoring the sacrum to its normal position, it is also true that these pulls have the effect of producing a further "floating" effect and so a very light pressure will somewhat move it and to some extent cause beneficial changes sufficiently to stop pain, and this can *always* be done. Pain will instantly stop – anywhere from any cause – if proper contact is made and held.

Such movement is *not* corrective, because as soon as "contact" is removed the pain will return unless a true correction of the sacrum has been made by a very light, accurate thrust, as will be explained in the Technic. In the latter case and providing no error is permitted, the pain will not return, and the trouble that caused the pain to begin will be better and will get well from that moment on.

The thrust indicated is by no means the heavy pound so long used by Osteopaths and Chiropractors. It is sufficiently heavy to "slightly spatter a cranberry" as taught in this book, and it is only by understanding the balance of this chapter that you will realize that it is far more effective, because it must be exactly right in contrast to the older "adjustments" of the same bone, which were usually "exactly wrong." We believe that it is only the tremendous ability of the body to adjust itself to new conditions that has prevented a large number of serious results from these older methods, because with *this* work the slightest error will produce such instant and such disastrous results that no other possibility remains.

The following illustration will show why this work, to be accurate, must be light. In the setting of heavy machinery that must be placed exactly so that its gears will mesh with others and driving rods will not bend, hydraulic jacks and steel and wood wedges are used until it is almost in place. Then, if the machinery is on the dotted line and must be moved to the heavy line, as shown in Figure 6, the entire machinery is held under stress, and especial stress is placed at the point marked 1. It can now be moved, though it weighs a hundred tons, with only a light tap of a hammer.

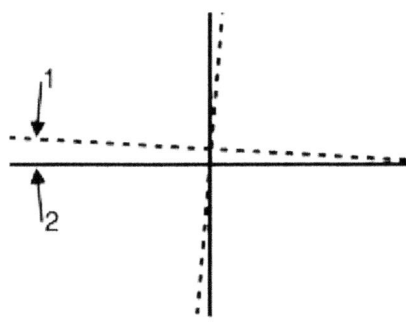

Figure 6

And this is the only way it can be set. If it is hit hard when under such stress, it will jump half an inch at a time, and in this illustration, that would reverse the diagram and then all the jacks would have to be replaced and special stress placed on the point marked 2. If the setting is not properly understood, this piece of machinery can be pounded back and forth and back and forth – with much loss of time and energy. If work is to be exact and accurate, it must be done intelligently and not in the slam away, hit-or-miss, methods of the past.

It is unanimously agreed that the human body is the most delicate and intricate mechanism on earth. Then begin to treat it as such and you will be amazed at the rapidity with which the body will recover and no longer be the sickest thing on earth.

The muscles act on the sacrum in the same way as the jacks act on the machinery that is being moved. Your contact is the jack that determines in what way that sacrum will move. Then remember that the lightest contact and the lightest drive (the tapping with the hammer) is all that is necessary if you wish to do a good job and not produce new distortions.

We have previously referred to the dangers of doing this work carelessly, ignorantly, or incorrectly, due to its high potential. This is a case of right being right and wrong being wrong. You will either take away distortion and strain or you will produce more of it. You will know you are right when you produce relaxation, and you will always be wrong if you produce any contraction anywhere in the body. Be sure you are not taking the strain from one part and placing it on another perhaps less resisting part. Now lay this book aside if you seriously consider working on someone, have that person undress to the knees if possible, spine bare at least, and see if you can trace all of this out while your patient is standing relaxed. If you cannot, then go back and read again.

As previously stated, the heaviest and most powerful muscles in the body are directly attached to the sacrum and the slightest deviation of the sacrum from its normal position puts one or more of these muscles under strain and makes it or them uncomfortable and causes pain. Just because these are the most powerful muscles of the body, if they are unable to cause the immediate correction of this deviation from normal, they commence transferring that strain to less and less resistant muscles throughout the body until from one slight slip, one minor distortion, we may find such widely spread troubles as a soft corn on a toe, a periodical and recurring headache with an inability to digest fat and in addition a symptom complex that will defy any diagnostician.

Every cell in the body, more every living cell and thing, is motivated all the time by selfish interest. There is no other motive force. You may give away the thing you so earnestly and bitterly struggled for, money or whatever it may be, but you will only surrender it when and as it suits your own selfish interest to do so. It may be possible for you to add more to your peace of mind or to your happiness to give money away than to keep it. In that case only will you give it away freely. There are occasions when pure nobility will show through the drab crust of men and they will sacrifice themselves for others as in shipwreck, etc., but because this violates the first law of nature, it never leads to the happiness of the one who makes the sacrifice.

The cellular structure of every living thing manifests exactly the same selfishness (the cold-blooded "fish" occupies a central position in the word), and muscles, which are groups of cells, must take on that characteristic, and do. Each muscle strives for rest; tries to shift its burden to some other; tries to secure its future without future effort, just as do people who are largely masses of muscle, all unmindful of that natural law, that what is left unused is soon removed. It is impossible to keep anything not constantly in service and so these muscles shed their loads, whether normal or abnormal, whenever possible upon those next less resistant on down the line exactly as people do.

Major-General Smedley Butler, after his experience in trying to clean up Philadelphia, is reported to have said in a speech that all the people should be divided into three groups. The first group consisting of those having $100,000 or over should have blue buttons, the possession of which would render them immune from arrest or trial for any crime, even murder or treason. While those having not less than $50,000 should have a white button and should be free to commit any crime less than murder or treason with immunity. While those having not less than $10,000 should have a red button and be immune from molestation for infractions of laws, ordinances, or rules up to but not including grand larceny. Those having less than $10,000 were not to be classed as people and were entitled to no consideration and should feel the full burden of all laws, all penalties, and all taxation.

He then startled his hearers by declaring that he was *not* joking. That it was now impossible to convict a member of one of the above groups of offenses listed and that the courts were jammed to the point of total inefficiency because of the futile effort to secure such convictions, and that his scheme would really react to the benefit of the masses who had less than $10,000 because they would be relieved of the tremendous costs of such courts, officers, and attaches, and they would be good, knowing there was no hope for them of evading the penalties.

Such government is sick government. Such a body politic is a distorted body and requires exactly the same kind of correction we teach for the human body in the present work, and it perfectly illustrates the transfer of burdens from the large and powerful to the smaller and less powerful, be they muscles or men. In government this leads to dis-ease in the shape of poverty, unemployment, social evils, graft, wars of aggression, and final oblivion, and all the treatments in the shape of treaties, pacts, agreements, and accords without, as well as tariffs, bureaus, subsidies, doles, etc., within are ineffective. In the body it leads to pain, unemployment, social evils, various complexes, incoordination, dis-ease, and death. And all the massages, poultices, liniments without, and pills, potions, and vaccines within are likewise unavailing.

Life Forces

All living matter has what we call life force. It is this only that distinguishes living forms, and the mystery of life is really the mystery as to why and how a cell materially similar in every respect to a nonliving cell can continually discharge energy, that is, continue to carry on the evidences of life. Every explanation or concept of the cause of disease and its correction that fails to take into consideration this great mystery must necessarily fail to explain or change smaller departures from normal than are required to reduce living matter to nonliving matter. That is, a system for the correction of disease, in order to be successful, must explain just what happens in such a case, why and how, and show the relation between this process and that which occurs in the human body when disease or death occurs and how it is controlled or improved by such method. It is this that we claim to explain, correct, and restore.

While we are not as yet able to state as facts all the essential points involved in the above, there is a wide knowledge being gradually accumulated, and the essential and important statements to follow are so positively known that only the conclusions drawn therefrom are subject any longer to question. We believe these conclusions justified both from the scientific and practical standpoint. If these conclusions seem to be reasonably logical and harmonious with past experience, previously known facts, and our present teaching, and our practical application produces the results naturally to be expected, and if in addition we find no evidence to the contrary, then we may safely assume that our teaching is correct, scientific, and beyond successful attack.

Any consideration of tissue depends for improved understanding of the subject upon a clear conception of just what is being discussed. The body is a vastly numerous group of cells, all essentially alike. Each possesses a nucleus, cytoplasm, and a cell wall. The chemical reaction in the nucleus is positive and acid, the cytoplasm negative and alkaline, while the cell wall is a fatty membrane resistant to the transfer of electrical energy. Within the cell wall are other fatty membranes, since each cell is in miniature a solar system, and each part of that system duplicates the structure as a whole and some state of electrical imbalance exists.

So long as this imbalance continues, the cell remains alive and able to carry on all of its marvelous activities. Just as soon as any chemical or electrical change occurs to disturb the acidity or positiveness of the plus elements or the alkalinity of the minus elements, just as anything reduces below normal the electrical or chemical imbalance, the cell becomes fatigued, then diseased, and if this disturbance continues until the imbalance is destroyed, the moment at which it is lost is the moment at which that cell ceases to live. The same is true of any group of cells making up a skin area, a vital organ, or the entire body, and the approach of death can be measured with accuracy by observing the gradually decreasing alkalinity of the fluids of the body. The instant at which the reaction of the blood crosses the line and ceases to be alkaline is the instant at which death occurs. This is not just a symptom of death. It occurs at that moment, and the reason is that the electrical energy, which is the life force, remains only so long as the chemical imbalance remains, and its tension exists in the exact degree that this chemical acidity and alkalinity persist.

Now we have previously noted that sarcolactic acid is produced in the cell during muscular activity. We have shown that it is removed in rest periods only. We have shown that muscles under constant abnormal stretch are physiologically in a state of contraction. We have shown that this condition invariably and necessarily exists when there is any distortion. We now come to the summary, which is that distortions, no matter how slight, necessarily produce fatigue and disease, acidity instead of alkalinity in the cytoplasm, loss of electrical potential, a loss of life force; and in proportion as these changes occur, death approaches.

It may be interesting in closing this chapter to refer to the fact that the electrical potential of a normal cell in a normal animal has been measured and is known to be on the order of

.8 microfarads* per square centimeter of surface. The thickness of the fatty wall surrounding such a cell has been measured and is known to be on the order of 4/10,000,000 of a centimeter. The total area of such cell walls in an ordinary human being has been calculated as approximately 98 square feet (Crile).

An ordinary electrical condenser of the oil immersion type, embodying exactly the same principles, is able to show only a small percent of the electrical efficiency of the condenser we ourselves are, yet it is dependent upon the maintenance of exactly the same condition, shows symptoms of failing power, and ceases to be useful, that is, dies, under exactly the same conditions.

---

*   Farad = The electrical unit of capacity whose symbol is C.
Volt = The electrical unit of electromotive force whose symbol is E.
Coulomb = The electrical unit of quantity = Ampere seconds = Q.
C = Q/E
Microfarad = 1/1,000 part of a farad.

CHAPTER V...THE SEXUAL LIFE

Preservation of the individual is the first law of nature.
Propagation of the species is the second.
Protection of the offspring is the third.

In accordance with the first, every reader of this volume must throw it aside without investigation of its principles and development of its values, or be intensely interested in its contents because everyone is sick or dis-eased more or less, and perfect, vital health is now within his grasp.

Happiness is the one and sole ambition of every person. Different roads are chosen by different people, but in the last analysis, it is this one word that describes the goal of humanity. There are different forms of happiness, thus accounting for the different roads followed. There are different conceptions of the material things necessary to happiness, but until a man or woman is certain of his own preservation, happiness is impossible as well as the secondary consideration. And since sickness, pain, and dis-ease are consciously recognized as a threat against this fundamental requirement, no one can possibly be happy so long as such conditions exist, and the amount and degree of happiness manifested is exactly proportionate to the seriousness of this threat.

So it is that chronic invalids sometimes are comparatively happy. They recognize no threat that is serious in their invalidism or any imminent change that will interfere with self-preservation. And so it is that the strong, vital person becomes a "bear" upon the least indisposition. The change from his usual vitality to his now lesser degree of it is to him a serious threat against his self-preservation. Besides, it requires far more effort in proportion to the available energy to keep a sick body alive than it does to keep a well body in top condition because of the enormous difference in the vital reserve, and the well man who becomes unaccountably sick must now turn an unaccustomed amount of energy into the business of getting well. He has already become conscious of lessened power and now this additional drain is of sufficient importance that he resents it. His resentment spreads to all about him. He blames everybody and everything as having a share in his disability and certainly he is cross, quarrelsome, difficult, etc., and remains that way until the disability lessens or disappears and he feels again competent to preserve self. Then once again he takes up the pursuit of happiness, he once again becomes jovial, pleasant, and an agreeable person.

This is true through the whole scale of human beings. The man who is accustomed to luxury becomes sullen and grouchy if his possessions are threatened, because to him these material things have become necessary to his happiness and almost necessary to his preservation. One accustomed to hardship would consider his future amply protected with the remainder of such possessions after a veritable calamity had occurred, which to the first man would reduce him to an impossible state.

But there is one thing common to all humanity that is the very next essential to happiness after health, and that is some means of expressing the creative power that marks man as the superior animal. To use it with satisfaction, man must use and learn to not abuse it in all of its expressions. The sex act is its most urgent, powerful, and productive or destructive form.

Happiness is impossible to any adult being without a normal sexual life – normal sexual expression – normal keenness of pleasure to both parties concerned. If any phase of this act is unsatisfactory to any party concerned, if there is no means of satisfying this desire, if there is any abnormality in its expression, then debility, degeneracy, etc., is to be expected, and happiness that is otherwise possible from every other angle is impossible so long as the disability lasts. This will become self-evident and immediately apparent upon a study of the technic embraced in this volume, for the areas occupied by the sexual organs must necessarily be the first involved in any distortion and the last to be completely restored to normal under correction. As long as any distortion exists in any body, just so long will some expression of the sex function be abnormal or there will be an abnormal lack of expression. This volume teaches just how to restore all these troubles in common with all others.

Let us anticipate the teaching of technic a little for the sake of making clear the next important point we wish to bring out. If all troubles have their origin in muscular tissue as already shown, then those we would be most conscious of would be found in the most muscular structures. This is true. For instance, a man may be very ill, yet quite comfortable on the whole, with tuberculosis, which very seldom attacks muscular structures, but he is never comfortable with even a slight attack of rheumatism, which seldom attacks any other than muscular structure.

Since all of the sex organs are particularly muscular and since their importance demands attention by their owners, anything wrong with them is soon impressed forcibly upon the consciousness. Thus irritations in early life and all too frequently in later years lead to masturbation and other abnormal sex expressions. Also, here as elsewhere, such conditions lead to constant inability to relax these muscular tissues, preventing rest and setting in motion the whole train of disturbances from a physiological aspect that we have already shown. If this condition continues over a long period of time, paralysis, partial or complete, is bound to occur.

Now, these contractured and overstretched muscles making up the organs in question can be felt, and the proper contact will instantly relax them. The proper correction will make that change permanent, thus restoring normal.

Since, as we have stated, these areas are the first to become involved by any distortion, the reason why we find sex troubles in practically every patient is self-evident. We have stated that no one is free from some degree of observable distortion, because no previous method was capable of correcting such conditions. We have shown that these distortions invariably produce sex troubles and now the reason why pregnancy is such a difficult time for so many women is apparent, as also is the terrible suffering and near approach to death caused by even a so-called normal delivery. Of course, such *tremendous elasticity* of muscular tissues as is then required is *impossible* in organs whose muscles have been in the abnormal contracted condition for long periods of time. As stated, the technic taught in this work *will correct all of this*. Our limited experience leads us to believe that we can ultimately render childbirth normal, painless, and completely safe.

Now again, distortion results from any load that exceeds the "elastic limit" of the individual, and the sex repression imposed by our code of morals by enforcing these repressions may produce such excessive loads and be itself directly responsible for the increasing of distortion. Especially is this true, because this involves the second most profound and deeply rooted powers of the body, and such distortions will produce widespread and disastrous results coming from here as from any other source. The sexual life begins at or before puberty. Our code of morals denies it any expression until adult years. This is *not conducive to health* and *is conducive to disease*. We are concerned with the eradication of disease, and it is therefore necessary to recognize this source of trouble to show its correction, to state that this one thing is sufficient in itself to explain all we have above mentioned and to direct the reader's thought to the removal of its causes. We are engaged in further researches in this and allied directions and are not yet ready to make any specific recommendations.

In closing this chapter, we wish to make one exception to the statement that no human being can be happy without normal sex expression, and that exception lies in those superior ones who have exhausted all the knowledge of life and living so obtainable and who have followed the twined serpents on the staff by turning their sex forces to a higher expression: a creative power much superior and a happiness more sublime. But these are more than human beings and the statement originally made stands true for the great masses of humanity.

CHAPTER VI...CHILDREN AND THEIR DISEASES

The abnormal sex life of the parents is the direct cause of difficult delivery, and this is the direct cause of childhood diseases, having robbed the child of a large part of its vital resistance. Now superimpose other strains beyond the "elastic limit" of the child, and we have the major causes of childhood diseases, all directly traceable to the strictures of society.

Hardly is a child born before it is forced to take food other than nature provided. Sometimes this results from the mother's inability, but this again goes back to the distortions and the sex habits of the parents. As soon as this is accomplished, the child is forced to conform to hours for food, sleep, play, etc., and then in rapid succession the control of the urine, the feces, and every other primal instinct of the race. At every point of control an unnatural condition is imposed upon it. Since only health is natural, any unnatural condition means ill-health and will never mean anything else. Here again we content ourselves in showing from a health standpoint just what is necessary and permit the student to make his own compromises. The advantage in stating all this is that if we know what is causing our ill-health, we no longer are helpless. We are then prepared for troubles whenever they arise and know what to do about them.

The abortive and suppressive methods of the medical doctor so generally used in these diseases are just like trying the abortive and suppressive levees in the Mississippi flood districts. When that water falls, the continued life of the districts involved depends upon their restoration to normal, and the river offers the easiest and only practical relief. Towns and districts just a little less able to protect themselves are burdened with what has become an excessive strain from the above, and they in turn throw up their own defenses, and so the unhealthy condition accumulates destructive force until in the lower reaches, the river, which usually and normally means the very existence of these districts, becomes so dangerous and intractable that within large areas all the normal activities of life are completely disjointed, and sometimes isolated communities pass out of existence.

A child develops colic, and the swelling and abundant vitality of that young body throws up its own defenses, the colic passes, leaving the levee behind it to interfere with traffic, and some slight inconvenience (constipation) is experienced and must be constant so long as the defense remains. The (rain) fall that produced the flood (of energy), which manifested in the child as colic, passes on, the child recovers, has a period of health, and then is sick again, disabled exactly as the next district down the river, but now the accumulated flood waters present a more serious problem, and the child has measles. Again the old levees are left after danger passes, and the eyes, nose, and throat are affected with a slight but permanent obstruction to traffic and are super-sensitive. And another period of apparent health while the flood waters are passing unsettled districts, then the child, as the next downriver district, is in trouble again – this time whooping cough with the same story repeated – then diphtheria, then scarlet fever, then adolescence and the age of typhoid, then early adult years and the flood has either carried away the child completely or little communities such as tonsils, adenoids, ear-drums, appendices, etc., have been destroyed. And so we go on through life experiencing ever more serious troubles and ever more serious impediments to free access, free functioning, free activities between the various elements of the flood valley and between the various parts of the human body until the end comes.

This is the chief reason why the reports of the Public Health Service (even though they are jammed to make them look well, like all medical propaganda) still show in regard to the widely heralded "lengthening of human life," that it really is no lengthening at all. In fact, human beings who pass forty-five live fewer years than before. Of course they do! They are now poisoned from birth and constantly encumbered with the old "levees" in increasing numbers. We quote from the *Reno Evening Gazette*, Friday, October 17, 1930:

"AVERAGE LIFE SPAN NOT INCREASED FOR AGED

"Adding ten years to the average span of human life is a notable accomplishment to the credit of the health agencies, especially when it is registered within the space of two decades, says the Providence Journal, which continues:

"That is what has been achieved in this country since 1910, according to a report of the United States public health service. The 'expectation of life' for an American baby at birth has been increased from forty-eight to fifty-eight years. That is a notable improvement in the infantile outlook.

"But the statistical proof of a ten-year increase in the American life span by no means demonstrates the fact of a similar extension all along the line, says the Journal. There is still an enormous wastage of health and life, as the federal authorities say, because of the prevalent failure to apply existing knowledge of sanitation and health. The infant's prospective span of life has been increased by ten years, but there has been no such extension of his chance after reaching the age of fifty. On the contrary, it is indicated that his 'life expectation' has been actually decreased. As compared with the man of that age twenty years ago, the man of fifty today faces a reduced prospect of reaching a 'ripe old age.'

"Substantially all the gain that has been made in health and longevity is entered on the ledger to the credit of juvenile life. The record of the elders steadily inclines to a red-ink deficit. 'Up to the present time,' says the report, 'the most significant advances in public health achievements have been manifested among the lower age groups. It is true, of course, that the great sanitary reforms, such as the filtration of water supplies, have remarkably diminished diseases of certain kinds among all classes and ages, but the actual saving of life has been most pronounced among children and infants.'

"The addition of ten years to the life span, in short, has been due to the great reduction of infant mortality and to the great advances made in the treatment of maladies particularly affecting children. The gain might have been materially larger had it not been for the marked increase in the degenerative diseases of middle age. The failure of medical science to work out a corresponding salvaging process with the higher age groups is due not to any shortcomings in the science but to the appalling weakness of the human equation. Infants and children are saved chiefly because they are helpless, and being helpless they have to submit to treatment."

Though the excuse is made in the above article that better results are had in children because they are forced to submit to treatment, no mention is made of the fact that these same children keep right on getting sicker. We know the only way to stop the accumulation of such flood water in later years, further down the valley, is to correct the condition at its source, and in the child that source is the uncontrolled and uncorrected results of the "fall." All methods that tend to abort or suppress abnormal conditions are like building these levees, and all medicines, toxins, antitoxins, etc., are such methods. This only leads to more and more illness in the future, and so we have more and more people in hospitals, sanitariums, rest-homes, etc., under "scientific care," yet they die and there are more and more sick people to fill their beds. This must indicate that more and more people are under treatment.

This then leaves the other excuse – the appalling weakness of the human equation. If science had no shortcomings, this weakness would by now be analyzed, understood, and corrected. Medical "science" *has* fallen short so far, because it has *not* solved the equation. And furthermore, they do not seem to be getting any closer to it.

Millions of dollars are spent for the sake of "science," and many interesting and important facts have been and are being discovered. But in spite of this, these facts are not being used to get you well and make it possible for you to get rid of all those little, as well as big and constantly recurring, illnesses that make man the sickest thing on the face of the earth, and constantly getting sicker. Now "science" or the most outstanding leaders of science are putting the blame back on you. They have done all they can. The following article also continues to twist statistics as brought out in the above quotation, and this appeared in the *Los Angeles Times* of October 14, 1931:

"NEW YORK, Oct. 14, (AP) – The way that hate, fear, worry, and jealousy have helped to choke off at 58 years man's hitherto rapidly increasing span of life was described to the American College of Surgeons tonight.

"The bank president worrying over business, the criminal suddenly stricken with fear, and the mother watching her sick child, all were pictured as doing the same injury to their health.

"This was discussed by two internationally known American physicians, Dr. George W. Crile of the Cleveland Clinic, and Dr. Charles H. Mayo of the Mayo Clinic of Rochester, Minnesota.

"Dr. Crile told the medical story of ravages of emotions of modern civilization. Dr. Mayo sketched remedies for ill health, which included newspapers as 'the greatest educating, thought-moulding enterprise in the world.'

"Both ascribed the recent increase in life to freedom from epidemics and world plagues of the past. Now, they said, comes a new and different phase when the individual must learn how to aid in his own healing, guided by the doctor."

We are to believe, according to this propaganda to the public, that never before in the history of the world have people experienced the above emotions until now – for the Bible records many instances of ripe old age of a few hundred years – and, if there were bankers, criminals, mothers, etc., before now, that they never had fears or worries. Yet we find on the oldest clay tablet of Babylon that these bankers, criminals, and mothers lived and carried on about the same then as now. And in the last paragraph you are told that now you must learn how to do your own healing, and that your doctor will guide you, though he has just told you that he has gone as far as he could and that his guiding leads to the grave. The doctors are using what knowledge they have in the following fashion, as appeared in an article in the *Los Angeles Times* (Oct. 13, 1931), which gives a striking example of the "scientific" way in which "cures" are made.

"BAFFLING HEART MALADY CURED
"Modern Life Results in Rapid Pulse
"Nerve Cutting Brings Back Normal Beat
"Operation Described for College of Surgeons

"NEW YORK, Oct. 13, (AP) – 'Soldier's heart' a baffling malady of modern high-pressure life, is reported cured by a recently perfected operation described to the American College of Surgeons tonight.

"Twenty of these new operations were discussed in a paper by their discoverer, George W. Crile, M.D., head of the Cleveland Clinic. Seventeen resulted in apparent cures.

"Soldier's heart was noticed, Dr. Crile said, during the World War. Its symptoms are rapid heart-beat, nervousness, and fatigue.

"'In the stress of civilian life,' his paper stated, 'many cases of this same disease are seen. Heretofore, there has been no effective treatment.'

"OPERATION BLOODLESS

"The operation is an almost bloodless and shock-free severing of the sympathetic nerves at their connection with the adrenal glands, a pair of diminutive, pancake-shaped, golden-colored endocrines near the kidneys.

"These two endocrine glands, Dr. Crile described as 'the power stations or brain of the sympathetic nervous system.' When they deliver an oversupply of energy to the sympathetic nerves, soldier's heart results."

"Science" has quit entirely looking for the factors that predispose to diseases or disorders in the human body. They do not now consider why these adrenals are stimulated to send out too much secretion. They recognize the fact that it does happen in some people. So they merely go inside and cut off the connection with the brain so that your body will no longer be conscious of trouble in the area complained of. And they call it a "cure." If you will read the little that is told about the adrenals in Chapter VIII of this book or read any authority on the subject, you will learn that if these glands can no longer respond to nervous stimuli, sent there in time of need, you will steadily grow into the condition described under poor functioning, which is as pitiable as that following the removal of the gonads. And "science" goes merrily on, maiming, torturing, and too frequently killing – while the people are kept complacent through the newspaper, "the greatest educating, thought-moulding enterprise in the world."

Right here, we wish it clearly understood that we are fully cognizant and aware of the abundant and valuable facts that have been developed in the Cleveland Clinic by Dr. Crile, the

Mayo Clinic by Dr. Mayo, the Massachusetts Poly-Clinic by Dr. Cabot, as well as Rockefeller Institute, etc. The pitiable thing is that they are not making the use of the facts for your own betterment that is possible, as we endeavor to show. If there had been no men as above and in the past, spending years in experimenting, some starving but still keeping on, this present work would have been unable to explain the cause of disease for the first time in our history. We wish to express our gratitude to that multitude of honest men. But when you see gifted, unusual, and capable minds as Crile and Mayo turn their eyes from all the facts they have found and tell you it is now up to you, that they can make no further use of what they know to help you, that it is now due to your emotional instability brought on by civilization (therefore could not occur in Babylon) – it is proof that they are either incapable or are deliberately refusing to make any constructive use of their knowledge for your benefit and comfort, as well as the future of your children.

The fact remains that they have conclusively proven that the living cell is immortal when supplied with the four essentials mentioned in Chapter II. And medical "science" has been increasingly unable to supply or apply these four essentials, so the human body grows weaker and weaker and dies within the same span of life, in spite of continuous improvement in food, recreation, sanitation, and general environment, which would of themselves, except for the offsetting effects of the continuous poisoning by vaccines and serums, destructive medicines and operations, reasonably have been expected to actually lengthen human life.

Aquarian-Age Healing is the first approach toward supplying and making logical use of these four essentials.

As previously stated, Fatigue and Disease are synonymous, and all knowledge carries out the statement. Then Rest and Rest-oration are synonymous. No disease is cured by any other method. No method is worthy of any consideration except it is conducive to this end. Some "old-fashioned" methods of handling these children's diseases do secure rest. No vaccine, toxin, antitoxin, or operation does. The technic taught in this volume will correct these strains and distortions and thus produce rest, and it still remains true that any pain can be instantly stopped and that acute troubles or painful conditions will get better from minute to minute under its proper application.

Watch your child when asleep. See if they are thoroughly and completely relaxed and quiet, breathing easily, deeply and regularly, with good color, breath, and body odor. If this condition exists, do not worry about that child "catching" any disease as long as the child continues to maintain this state. This does not mean that you should unnecessarily expose the child to any infection just to see if he will "catch" something, for even though no one knows just what it is, there is a principle of infection, and no good can come of such foolishness as exposing a child to measles just to have it over with.

But if you see a child all curled up in a ball or stretched in unnatural positions, and especially if you find it on its knees with the elbows and face in the bed, or twitching, moaning, tossing, or kicking, you can be sure there is something wrong, and the body is making a great effort to correct it. Failing that correction, the child will soon be ill. As soon as you see this, be sure that your child receives the correction it requires, as taught in this book, and all will be well. Threatened disease will be avoided, certainly and surely.

If you fail to do this and the child continues to develop some "childhood disease," you will have only yourself to blame for it, and if the trouble proves to be one of the acute infections such as diphtheria or scarlet fever, the serious after-effects will exactly follow in the areas affected, that is, those areas that were subject to the greatest strain, as indicated by the posture you paid no attention to. These areas now are the seat of chronic disease and represent "accumulated fatigue," which will rob the child of the ability to get that kind of sleep which is so typical of the healthy child and which adults so often envy. Even after all the above has happened, it is still possible to restore the child by persistently following the instructions herein.

CHAPTER VII...EYES, EARS, NOSE, MOUTH, AND THROAT

There is probably no part of the body so much abused at big prices as these areas. All sorts of "specialists" on these areas are commanding high prices for continuous operations that seem always to be only the introduction to some other operation. It is our sincere desire to state only facts as we know them and to give all credit where credit is due, but in these cases in particular, we have never seen a cure follow any of these operations on any of these organs, and the disappointing, not to say disgraceful, results that we have seen would fill a larger book than this one.

When advised to have such an operation – DON'T.

The above, of course, has nothing to do with the repair of direct injury from accidents. Broken noses and jaws must be set, the same as broken legs, and the job is sometimes so complicated that the best result is none too good. Even in these cases the application of the teachings herein will offer instant relief and greatly assist the cure.

Trouble in the above-mentioned areas is strictly muscular in origin: a statement as radical as can well be imagined, especially to the layman. The occulist, optometrist, physician, in fact the doctor of any school, will be forced to admit the following statements to be true:

Strabismus (crossed eyes), a strictly muscular trouble.

Myopia (near sight), a strictly muscular trouble.

Hypermetropia (far sight), a strictly muscular trouble.

Astigmatism (fuzzy sight), a strictly muscular trouble and glasses will never *restore* it to normal.

The above will meet no resistance. All doctors are agreed on these points, but what about:

Retinal hemorrhage, a strictly muscular trouble? If not, why does it attack only a very small area of the eye, frequently only one eye? There is a wrong muscular condition at the point of attack, else the retinal artery would not break down just there. People who suffer this trouble seldom have apoplexy, which is the name of an exactly similar trouble when the hemorrhage occurs in the brain. In either case, muscular fibers in the walls of an artery fail because of local fatigue.

But there are many other troubles such as glaucoma, iritis, choroiditis, corneal ulcer. What about them? In each case, a strictly muscular trouble. In the case of glaucoma, continuous contraction of the muscles in the eyeball prevents the normal removal of the humors of the eye, permitting them to accumulate and sometimes cause such tremendous pressure inside the eyeball that it bursts. Real pain accompanies this condition. And so on, with every trouble of the eye. Each is a separate, definite, and strictly muscular trouble in the last analysis.

The ears are exactly to the same extent subject to muscular troubles. There is nothing else. Even the entry of foreign bodies into the eye or ear results frequently in troubles called by all sorts of names, depending on the exact symptoms most prominent, but each one in its last analysis is a muscular trouble and nothing else. This includes all deafness, vertigo, and so forth. We cannot be too plain in our statement.

The nose with the antrum, sinus and mastoid cells, polypi, adenoids, catarrhal conditions, etc., will not require your sprays and douches, the caustics and antiseptics so widely prescribed, advertised, and used. The ears also should be left alone. "Never put anything in the ear that is smaller than your elbow," is good advice. And the throat should not have its mucous membranes hardened, thickened, and ultimately destroyed by the constant use of the "remedies" so widely recommended. There are many reasons for this, but one alone is sufficient. By the use of such remedies, you relieve the body of looking after its own defenses, and the old natural law again works: what is not used is removed.

The tonsils and adenoids especially should not be tampered with. They are the only part of the lymphatic system that normally contacts the outer air, and though we do not have a very clear idea of their purpose, the fact that they can be returned to full usefulness again should cause their preservation as a valuable indication of deeper troubles early enough to avoid serious disturbances in tissues whose vital function is better understood. A well-known doctor of Johns Hopkins publicly stated that he never again would remove a tonsil, and this after the statement that he had taken out more of them than any other living man. He said he had removed "literally bushels of them."

And now we attempt to state the fact regarding dentistry, another branch of medicine only a few years ago adopted and taken into the fold, and already we have an enormous number of "specialists" in this work, and again the patient is almost, if not quite, always worse off after the "specialist" is through. A hole in a tooth needs filling – "Maybe." The hole cannot get there without something having destroyed the resistance of the enamel, and that is the only part of the tooth that is equipped to resist wear and destruction. Its business is to protect the softer structures beneath, and if it has a hole in it, that tender and nonresistant part of the tooth will soon be likewise destroyed.

Even dentists will agree that no tooth should ever be pulled out, but because they do not know the fundamentals, not even the first steps in improving teeth – and this is so true that many a dentist will deny that it can be done, they take them as they find them, they fill them as long as they can, they inlay them, then crown them or cap them, and the next thing they pull them, or rather some "specialist" does. Then to fill the hole where the tooth was, they pull one or two good ones on the opposite side so as to "balance" the bridge and finally turn you loose without the ability to chew your food. You go along for a while, finally get them all out "to be done with it," and get a pair of plates (dentures in polite society), and find out that you can chew less than ever.

There are comparatively few people over forty who have not suffered a large part of the above, especially if they have had the advantages (?) of city life and city doctors, but these are the people who had pretty even and pretty good teeth to begin with. If the dentist had a chance at you and your teeth were just a little crooked, as is normal to some types (see Chapter VIII), he induced you to have that condition corrected. Thousands of children are running around today with mouths full of screw jacks, guy wires, and other insane devices, all meant to loosen the teeth in their sockets so that they can be forced to take different positions. If this is successfully accomplished, pyorrhea later on is almost certain, and a new "bite" is positively certain, for the teeth will not change their shape or size for all the dentists and specialists that play around on them. Then, a little off here, a little off there, a lot off somewhere else, and the enamel that was meant to last a lifetime is to a large degree destroyed at once. This is surely "conservative methods" with a vengeance.

Never permit anything of this sort!

In all these areas DIET is just as important as with diseased conditions in other parts of the body. The proper diet will change the character of teeth as well as their color, will definitely change the condition of eyes, ears, nose, or throat, and all of these requirements will be provided for if our chapter on diet is understood and carefully followed.

We are writing only "pointers." If each of these subjects in this book was exhaustively explained, we would have to write a library and no one would read it. You must do your own thinking. You can do your own thinking, and it is surely worthwhile to do your own thinking.

In all of these areas, the proper application of this technic will give gratifying results. Just try it.

CHAPTER VIII...THE DUCTLESS GLANDS

This chapter is included only because of its wide general interest at the present time. There is little original work represented, the entire chapter being merely a copy of notes accumulated over a number of years: many writers, many sources. Since the notes were not accumulated for publication, due credit cannot be given to each author, the sources having been destroyed after the notes were made and no record of such sources kept.

It had been entirely unnecessary to develop any particular study of these glands because we find that they respond just the same as all other parts of the body to a proper application of the technic, and any abnormalities listed in this chapter as a result of glandular trouble will be rapidly corrected.

The ductless glands, otherwise called the glands of internal secretion or the endocrines, comprise the following:

SPLEEN: Has to do with the antibodies and corpuscle production. It has been said that a normal spleen makes contagious or infectious diseases impossible.

THYMUS: Disappears or is greatly reduced in size at puberty, or if persistent aside from other marks of inferiority, it produces irregular, pearly, translucent teeth, scalloped or crescentic on the bite; central incisors large; lateral incisors small, underdeveloped, or missing. Retards the development of the sex apparatus until the body is well grown.

THYROID: A regulator, tending to speed up the function and metabolism of the body. If poor in function, besides other marks, produces poor, soft, decaying, and widely separated teeth. If in good function, produces good, small, regular, and glistening teeth.

PITUITARY: Has important influence on muscle, tendon, and nerve development and use. If poor in function, produces malformed, crowded, and irregular teeth. If good, produces large, broad, square, and regular teeth.

PINEAL: Governs sex organ development.

PARATHYROIDS: Important in calcium metabolism. If poor, produces poor, soft, and brittle teeth.

SUPRARENALS, sometimes called ADRENALS: Furnish the stimulus for outbursts of energy necessary in fighting or running away. If good, produces hard, strong, but yellow teeth, especially the canines or "eye-teeth."

GONADS: The testicles in men, the ovaries in women. The glands of chief importance in the primary and secondary sex manifestations.

COCCYGEAL BODY: Whose function has not been discovered, or at least information concerning which has not come to hand.

Sometimes the pancreas is included because of an internal secretion, but this organ as well as the liver and kidneys, which are sometimes included as well, are not truly organs of *internal* secretion, all being provided with ducts. The mere fact that they have some such secretion does not set them apart from all the other structures of the body, because we believe there is in the same sense internal secretion from every part and cell in the body.

In addition to the above, the following may be interesting. The thyroid, when active, produces a beautiful body with fine skin and hair, usually wavy. The structure of such a body is rather tall and slender, but with unexpected power in its grace. If the thyroid fails, the anterior section of the pituitary becomes larger. The thyroid enlarges and diminishes in size and function in sympathy with the gonads. Goiter cases, in common with other diseases, show sexual troubles, but usually with more definiteness.

Thyroid deficiency produces ugly bodies. The features are coarse, the eyes dull, the nose is broad and flat, the teeth poor, hair scant and coarse, the skin thick and dry, the stature short, the hands and fingers short, thick, and cold, the nails brittle, the pulse, temperature, and blood pressure low. They are languid and tired, have no interest in life and no power to create one. They are frequently the victims of dementia praecox.

The pituitary, when active in men, usually produces a body over six feet tall and beautifully formed, which never gets fat, although sometimes a short, stubby, round, but hard and durable body. When this gland is inactive, the body is soft and fat, especially below the waist, of poor quality, and tired. The mentality shows the same lack of power, and these people are subject to diabetes, impotence, epilepsy, homosexuality, mongolism, etc. They are small in every way and are frequently in police courts.

The pineal is most active in childhood, gradually losing its activity until it calcifies at about thirty years. It holds back sex and maturity, physical and mental, until the body reaches its growth. Tuberculosis of this gland has been known to cause complete maturity in the sex organs even in very young children.

The parathyroids are usually present in pairs and are found in connection with the thyroid, but sometimes those of one side are entirely missing, and in these cases, if the glands from the other side are taken out, the patient dies. They control the lime metabolism, and if they are deficient, the bones and teeth are poor and soft and the general development is deficient.

The suprarenals, when functioning well, produce a body with hard and durable structure, but not very beautiful. The hair is thick and coarse, the skin dark and freckled, the teeth are good but yellow, the head round and hairy, the face broad, the blood pressure high. These people are aggressive, pugnacious, progressive, optimistic, and excitable. In women, there is usually a masculine tendency; they are the comic strip "suffragette" of a few years ago and those who are "just as good a man as you are, Junga Gin," and are usually lacking in ovarian function.

If these glands (suprarenals) are deficient in function, the body is short and obese and lacks all of the qualities listed above as resulting from a plentiful secretion from these glands. These people are usually the victims of insomnia or think they are, for they are asleep while walking around and awake while asleep. Their level of positiveness is so near their sleep level that there is no real demarcation line.

The gonads appear to be the regulators of the entire endocrine system and the brain. They are necessary in normal function to control the development and the activities of the entire body, and any removal of these glands in early life means infantilism, nothing less and always. If functioning properly, the individual has or will have a strong sex nature, big bones, big voice, big strength, big endurance, and a "big heart." They are vital people, "personalities," and do things. If functioning poorly, naturally the reverse is true and the person is one to be pitied, because the extreme condition does not result except through surgical interference, and in these cases, even this technic is limited. For although the body has amazing powers of adaptation and all of the powers will be used in their full effectiveness if the corrections herein taught are properly applied, even to the extent of changing materially the characteristics of a mature body, it is impossible to entirely compensate for organs or glands that are missing.

The products of these glands of internal secretion are most powerful and have marked effects on the body, even when greatly diluted, as is shown by Jerome Alexander in his *Colloid Chemistry*. He states, "The posterior lobe of the pituitary yields to the blood a very potent hormone.... Krogh estimates that this hormone is effective in less than one part in one hundred million, while Abel has isolated a purified hormone said to be effective in one part in 18,750,000,000."

The ductless glands seem to hold the riddle of heredity, and since they can be so greatly influenced by the work we teach, it seems likely that even hereditary traits can be and will be considerably modified thereby.

CHAPTER IX...PSYCHOLOGY

Living is a Positive State.
Thinking is a Positive State.
Concentration is a Positive State.

All the processes of living depend upon action. Action requires power, and the exercise of power is the most positive thing that man is capable of, and so far as the finite mind can imagine, it is also the highest and most positive attribute of God. It is the God force in man, the wider creative power, that makes him the superior animal.

The following may not be in line with the teachings of some "psychologists," but in sleep the brain has been observed, the liver has been observed, the facts are scientifically established, and no argument may be well-based in ignorance of these findings.

Sleep is a Negative State.

It is the *only* negative state normal to man. Any other negative state induced is a deliberate sacrifice of the highest powers of man and leads of itself directly to its ultimate form, death and disintegration. But sleep is only relatively negative to the positive state that preceded it, which is not true of the other negative states. If there were no other reason than the above for warning against resort to faith cures, this one alone should be sufficient, but the negative state also attracts other disabilities too varied and numerous to discuss here, all of which are destructive in effect.

Thinking is a positive action, and as long as thinking persists, it is impossible to induce a negative state. Hypnotists know this. Concentration is one of the prerequisites to thought. Therefore, it is impossible to concentrate on a negative subject unless you can make it positive to yourself. This thinking mind is not open to "suggestion." In this work the patient *must* concentrate and *must* think. There is no "psychology" used or needed.

Sleep and disease are negative states; therefore it is impossible to produce either the one or the other by thought or concentration.

"The Silence" is a Negative State.

Contemplation is a Negative State.

Receptivity is a Negative State.

In all of these, the mind is deliberately placed in a negative state. You "await," and so you may in these states induce sleep or disease. Or if faith, another negative state, is also present, you may be "cured" of disease, as it has already been shown that where pain is not present in the consciousness, there is no *dis-ease in the consciousness.* This freedom from the consciousness of disease will continue so long as your own negativity shuts out your positive thought. Such a lack of consciousness of disease does not mean that the disease process is stopped, bettered, or corrected. It does continue and must continue no matter how great the faith, no matter how great the negativity, and will produce death because the distortion that caused the disease will sooner or later destroy the vital powers of the organism exactly as in the case of the diabetic who does not know he is sick. As soon as consciousness is manifest, then we see reactions to things that might be expected to cause pain, and reactions of things that might be interpreted by such consciousness as disease.

Thus, plants will show definite reactions similar to those manifested by creatures in which a brain can be demonstrated as soon as they are subjected to destructive forces, such as cutting or crushing of their fruit or branches. This interesting work has been carried on principally by Dr. Bose, who received the award of the Nobel Prize for his original work. These reactions are absent if the damage is done while the plant is under the influence of deadening drugs, just as they are in men. Thus, there is no pain and no consciousness of disease.

We must carefully distinguish between the actual and the conscious presence of disease. Tuberculosis, nephritis, diabetes, atrophy of the liver, to mention only a few, even various very evident paralyses, cause no active *consciousness of disease* in the mind, yet it would not be contended that there was no disease. But none of these diseases is PRIMARY. They are all SECONDARY, and the primary or acute disturbances which gave rise to them were all marked by conditions in which the sufferer actually had disease in the consciousness because of painful impressions, and these were the earliest symptoms of disease.

The question may still arise whether sleep really is a negative state and, if so, how it can be that it is only in this condition that man repairs and restores his body and his energies and, if this is not the case, how then can we maintain our basic idea that exhaustion is the only cause of death.

Let us suppose we have a perfectly normal human being. Every cell in his body is functioning at its highest abilities, and then we would say such a man was functioning at 100% level. The chances are that our best average level is about 80%, and on this scale and just for the sake of illustration, we could say that a 50% level means serious illness and bed, 25% will mean death, and 0% will mean disintegration of the body. There is still left the atomic energy in the atoms that made up that body, and it has been calculated that the atomic energy contained in one-half glass of water is sufficient to drive the largest Atlantic liner a round trip to Europe. This energy is not available to what was once the organized man, so we are able to know that 0% of energy in the organism means disintegration. Because of the fact that hair and nails grow after death, that all organs do not "die" at the same moment and other facts, we believe we are fairly close to the truth in stating that 25% of energy means death. Our estimate that 50% means serious illness and bed is very rough, but probably not far from the truth, and our estimate of 80% level as the best average is generous.

A disability that forces a man to lie down when a certain degree of illness is present is itself nature's best provision for his cure. It enforces a certain degree of rest. It relieves him also of the necessity to resist the forces of gravity, thereby conserving a tremendous amount of energy. This most frequently happens in the so-called self-limiting diseases, as we all know, and the process is one of first removing the excess load and then repairing the damaged structure, as we state in our first group of concepts. If this repair process can be carried on when the body is functioning at somewhere between 75% and 50% levels, then it would seem that the natural and best level for such activities would exist during normal sleep when the body has dropped easily and quietly from its 80-100% level of positiveness to say a 70% level of positiveness, which in this case is relative negativeness and probably the normal sleep level. This idea is supported by the fact that when the body dropped in its average function from the 80% level to near the 70% level, restlessness usually begins. That is, the change from positive to less positive is not sufficiently great to cause the patient to lose consciousness, and he awakes from such sleep as he has gotten complaining of being just as tired as before, or more so, and of having spent a sleepless night. If this is true, then sleep IS a *relatively* negative state.

The above does not take into consideration the "miraculous cures" of the great healers of history. We do not attempt here to analyze, classify, dispute, or acclaim miracles, and this book teaches nothing concerning them. The purpose of this book is to reduce to scientific facts, reasonable processes, tangible procedures, and complete methods, all that is required to get any sick body well, and does that so successfully that no discussion of or belief in miracles, or even these teachings, is necessary to a cure.

Do the work herein taught with understanding, accuracy, and often enough to correct the distortion present, and you will agree with the authors that, though the day of miracles may be past, no one need regret the passing.

CHAPTER X...DIET

There is no cure in dieting. It is sometimes necessary to adhere to a very rigid diet for a given period of time. Acidosis must be controlled and sometimes controlled quickly.

Diet helps. There is always a need to nourish the body, but the body is not nourished by the food eaten. It is nourished only by the food properly digested and assimilated. Food of poor quality or poorly selected cannot be called a normal diet, but everyone must have this normal diet and in sufficient quantities if he is to be a normal person. No amount of correction will take the place of food, exactly as no amount of lying in bed without rest will restore a fatigued body.

Given a normal diet, every person who has obtained the correction taught in this volume will gradually approach whatever weight and strength are normal to that person. People are not all alike, just as horses are not all alike, and even though we deliberately mix breeds in people and keep the breed straight in horses, we do get in spite of that some persons who are light, fast, alert, and sensitive like Arabians and the reverse: heavy, slow, calm, and dependable like a Clydesdale. It is absolutely impossible to feed an Arabian like a Clydesdale without making him sick, and it is the same with men; and you do not change the type in the one case any more than you do in the other. No matter what your own classification is, develop that to its best powers and be happy.

There is a man, a former patient of Dr. Hurley's, who is six feet seven inches, whose body is very well-proportioned and durable, who is so much above the average that he was questioned particularly about his family history. It developed that for over 300 years no male of the direct line has been less than six feet three inches tall and that the famous regiment of the English Palace Guards, where unusual height is the first qualification, has in all that time never been without a representative of the family. If we are what we eat, why did not large numbers of people whose environment and consequently whose foods were similar develop a like height? And why, with all the changes in diet that the passage of years (to say nothing of centuries) brings, was the general stature of this family unaffected?

Diet will not change nor will anything else change the heritage of man, but proper diet and the near approach to perfect functioning as it is understood today, made possible by this work, will bring all persons to their best functional level. The normal diet requires sufficient protein to make good the building needs of the body, sufficient carbohydrate to make good the energy needs of the body, and sufficient fat to furnish the fuel to sustain it. In addition, it must have an overabundance of mineral salts, and this will guarantee sufficient vitamins. After all that is provided, there is still required a sufficient bulk of *non-digestible* and non-putrefying foods to give the peristaltic action of the bowel something to squeeze upon and to carry away by absorption the highly poisonous wastes that are constantly being poured into the intestinal canal due to the breaking down processes the body continually undergoes. The last requirement demands at least four pounds of food daily, but NOT its equivalent in nutritive value.

We know that a man who is functioning perfectly can remain so for continued periods of time if he has nothing to eat but grass and bark. We know that a man on the trail with a dog team in the coldest of weather, and even in the far north, usually eats three or four slices of barely-heated bacon and two or three small flapjacks with a tin of black coffee twice a day and makes remarkable distances on it. But we know, too, that at the end of the trail, seldom longer than ten days, he reaches camp and eats all of the foods his body needs; he usually just eats for several days. Then, too, on the trail or in the camp, he is never without whiskey. This does not mean that he drinks it to excess. Transportation limitations make it too valuable to waste, but he uses a little of it all the time.

We know that all carnivorous animals take first the blood and the entrails of their kill and only afterwards commence on the muscular tissue, if at all. Natives who are forced to live on exclusively a meat diet do the same. When white men, arriving amongst such natives, are too "particular" to eat this way, they soon become ill and recover only if and when they adopt the native way.

We know the "Kronprinz Wilhelm" could have kept the high seas and possibly changed the history of the World War if her medical officers had kept the foods they jettisoned – and they jettisoned most of what they took off captured ships – but they did not know that meat, potatoes, bread, cheese, cream, butter, champagne, without a great abundance of fruit and vegetables, will kill the strongest man. The whole crew became ill. Not enough men were left to operate the vessel. She was forced to abandon her war activities and put into the Potomac River, and all the American medical authorities failed to help those ill. Finally, a layman named McCann, one-time assistant to Dr. Wiley and a dietician of ability, went aboard as a reporter, stayed in spite of all efforts to displace him by the medical authorities, and caused the rapid recovery of all these sick men by administering vegetable juices exclusively.

We also know that a man who is not functioning perfectly may starve to death even though he has the best foods of all the world to choose from or eat. We know that a man in ordinary condition can fast with no food but water and do considerable work for periods of up to forty or fifty days without damage. We know that if this same man is lost in the mountains or suffers fear of death from any cause, he may show all the evidences of starvation in only a few days.

And the above and its like are about all that is positively known in relation to diet, and food chemistry is changing so rapidly that we can place no positive reliance on most of it. Yet, there are some well-established facts that we add here because of their possible value in certain cases.

Thompson seedless grapes are usually of value in conditions where too much water accumulates in any part of the body (dropsical conditions). The patient may eat three or four pounds of these a day and nothing else with good results.

Red beets are usually valuable in rheumatic conditions. They are not useful as an exclusive diet.

Vinegar is frequently prohibited in the very cases where it may be of value: where imperfect fat digestion is the trouble.

Potatoes are an excellent food if used in a balanced diet. They furnish a larger percentage of potassium than any other common food, and potassium is an essential element for brain function particularly. Many cases of failing memory will be improved if potatoes are eaten or eaten more freely.

Pineapple will be found to help all stomach conditions accompanied by sore throat and should not be eaten in large quantities or alone at any other time except in countries where it grows.

Tomatoes are a very valuable food as intestinal disinfectant. It is easy to eat too many.

Nuts, oils, and whole wheat make a combination that will replace meat and meat products, but meats must not be withdrawn for long periods from the dietary without the substitution of *all* of these.

Greater endurance is built upon a strictly vegetable diet than upon a meat or mixed diet, but the general powers, the positiveness, of an individual are built and maintained best upon a mixed diet or one in which the above substitutions have been intelligently made.

Watermelon or pears will often alleviate stubborn constipation if eaten plentifully and alone.

Starches and commercial sugar are readily convertible into energy and are thus valuable, but so far as refined sugars are concerned, their value stops there. The energy must have other materials to support the effort, and if they are not taken with the sugar, the body loses them out of its reserve. Devitalized sugar is not a food at all. No concentrated foods of any kind will sustain life. They are permissible only as emergency rations and for very short periods of time. No one can live upon them and maintain health or condition. Malted milks with egg and other similar mixtures fall within this grouping and will destroy the benefits of a proper dietary adhered to during the balance of the day. The soda fountain lunch is so destructive that we would rather have a patient under our care eat nothing at all at that time rather than a soda fountain lunch. We have no objection to a dish of ice cream or a soda as an occasional small treat.

Lima beans, dried preferably, furnish a larger percent of alkaline ash than any other usual food of the American dietary.

Whole wheat flour produces a larger percent of acid ash than white flour, making it less desirable from this standpoint, but is still the best because of its much larger food value.

People who are ill will, as a rule, do better on an exclusively fruit diet (and the more raw the better) than any other. For more detailed instruction, see any good book on diet, such as *The Normal Diet* by Sansum (Mosby & Co., St. Louis, MO) at any bookstore.

We have found that we ourselves do better when we eat about as follows. The practice of this method is hard work, both mental and physical, added to which are the large responsibilities assumed. We need plenty of food, as you will see.

Breakfast

Not less than two pounds of juicy fruit, raw and natural, per person.

Lunch

A large serving of two freshly cooked leafy or juicy vegetables, a large raw salad, one or two slices of whole wheat bread, a little butter, and salad dressing.

Dinner

Soup

Meat

Salad

Potatoes plus one other vegetable

Whole wheat bread

Milk, coffee, or tea

Dessert

And nothing between meals.

When you see a patient who is too fat or too thin, too hard or too soft, and so on, do not try to correct by diet. More harm has been done by such methods than will ever be known. The body knows its own requirements far better than you do. Many will deny the truth of the above without trial. Those who try will find the statements exactly true. The body is an organism, and if there is disease in one part of it, there is some measure of disease in every part of it, because the body must function as a whole, and to function harmoniously or to be in a state of health, every part of it must be in that same state. Any part of the body that fails to do that, or that shows excessive fat or lack of it and so on, is destroying the health of the body to a very exact, though as yet unknown, degree.

To illustrate with a man who is thin and hard. It is generally stated that this man should take things easy, rest much, eat foods high in nutritive values, stop worrying, play at quiet games, and put on weight. Let us see. It is well known that this type of man has an "excessive" secretion from the adrenal glands. This is the reason he is active, belligerent, forceful, capricious, swift, tough, unstable emotionally, impulsive; why he likes active muscular play and work, sleeps little, rests little, and relaxes never at all. Force this man to change his habits of life, and that secretion that kept him going, that forced him to keep on going, will poison him and ultimately kill him because its energy must be expended, and you have stopped the expenditure.

Note how such people are often sick after great unexpressed anger. The diet usually recommended will also kill them, as they cannot digest or assimilate it. You must find and correct the thing that makes this "excessive" secretion necessary, and immediately it will be no more. The person will then commence to function normally, will require and secure the rest and sleep he so sadly needs, will enjoy the quiet relaxation so desirable for him, and as a result will lose the over-hardness and the leanness; in other words, will get well. Any other way ends in disappointment always, even death sometimes.

There is now and always has been since diet commenced to occupy the minds of people an insistent demand for a set diet for this or that condition and for this or that patient. It is utterly impossible to satisfy any such demand from a scientific standpoint. Faddists can do it. The demand springs from those who are unwilling or unable to study the facts for themselves, and these are the people who will never follow any diet in any case. They want to get well, but not enough to do the necessary things.

A diet in which you are given exactly so much of this and so much of that for each meal, and then have the process repeated for the next meal, can be laid down only if and when the patient is under the most rigid institutional care, for it presupposes that nothing will be taken into the body that is not included in the dietary, that everything that is so included will be taken, and that this state of affairs will continue without a break. It presupposes, in addition, control of the habits of every kind, rest, exercise, and so on, and upon all of this, by the aid of chemical and physical tests carried out carefully and persistently together with direct observation of the patient, such a diet can ultimately be arrived at, and it is not possible in any other way whatsoever.

The information given in this chapter, though short and condensed, is very much to the point, and anyone who will study it and then REGULATE his habits accordingly will find that, with the correction as taught being carried out, he will make rapid and constant improvement, and by watching carefully the effect of minor changes in the diet adopted, he will soon correct what slight error is certain to arise.

CHAPTER XI...EXERCISE

In our chapter on psychology, we assumed that the level upon which our body manifests in waking hours and in health is probably on the average of about 80% of its maximum and that 70% is its approximate level during healthful and refreshing sleep. It seems to be true that this 70% level does not change greatly in ordinary "health" but that the spread increases as the "awake level" goes up, so that sleep becomes ever more restful and refreshing. Now, if the awake level can be raised, more and better rest is assured. This technic does raise this level, and we have not yet found its maximum ability in this direction, but there are other ways of doing it, and one of the most important is exercise. The reason is obvious.

The functioning level is a direct reflection of the similar level in the cell. This is measured by the relative acidity and alkalinity or by the electric potential, as was before explained. This in turn depends upon oxidation, and the rate of oxidation depends upon demand. Nature's law that what is not used is soon removed has also been referred to, and so no matter what your present rate of oxidation, disuse will lower it, full use will raise it. "Unto him who hath, more shall be given, and to him who hath not, that which he hath shall be taken away."[3] The full

---

[3] Paraphrase of *Matthew 25:29* of the Christian Bible.

use of the muscular power of the body is the most direct, speedy, and certain means of increasing oxidation, as anyone can prove by the heavier breathing and greater intake of air upon even slight exertion.

The subject of air intake somehow fails to receive the attention it really should have, due to its prime importance. If a person is a little constipated for a day or two, he is usually disturbed about it and resorts to radical methods for changing it, frequently leaving a worse condition fundamentally than before. If the urine is known to be even slightly abnormal, these same people will resort to what frequently are dangerous methods of destroying the abnormal indication, reckless of its long-time effects. If they fail to eat exactly on time, they suffer headaches and other discomforts and resort again to destructive medicines, forgetting or ignorant of the fact that hunger should and normally does increase the body powers so as to enable the animal to make what unusual effort is necessary to obtain food. If they are thirsty, they again suffer discomfort and will drink anything, even the slush that is called soda-pop, far more destructive than any wine, beer, or any good liquor.

But they will allow their breathing to become shallower and fainter from day to day, week to week, year to year, and do nothing about it until they actually lose the "breath of life," and it is said they died a "natural death." It is a terrible misconception. They died by suicide as surely as if they had hanged themselves. The only difference is that the agonies of strangulation did not come upon them as suddenly in one case as in the other. They experienced all these pains, but they were strung out over a period of months or years and were never associated with the slow strangulation that was occurring.

Man can work hard without any food but water for days and weeks, as before stated. He can do without water, if necessary, for hours at a time even in hot weather and at hard work. But he cannot do without air for even a few minutes either at work or at rest. Everyone knows this, but hardly anyone pays any attention to it, probably because air is the one thing the body needs which it secures in some measure without conscious effort. Certain it is that what is easily obtained is lightly prized. But too much food will ruin good digestion, too much water will make you totally unable to produce any work of any kind (ask a farmer when to water a horse or a garden), but too much air is impossible to obtain. The more you take of it, the faster you use it. The more you can take of it *and the greater your output of energy*, the higher your functioning level.

No patient will ever die of acute lobar pneumonia if you can induce or force him to take six deep breaths when he first is sick and drive them down so deep that the air *passes the place that hurts*. This is a painful process and will require all the energy the patient can muster, but it will break up the developing pneumonia process, and if it is at once followed by proper application of this technic, your patient will be out of danger and bed in a few hours. Without the breathing, the same result will be had under this technic but in a slightly longer time.

No exercise is of any value unless it does produce increased demand for air. If you have so little energy that you cannot work and just play around with it, you had better use what small energy you do possess in getting your distortion corrected, or failing that, getting your affairs in shape for someone else to handle. You will need that someone soon enough, for though a person is too sick to move, he can still increase his breathing, and even this is a sufficient start.

This is the reason why *active* outdoor games are so productive and why golf is the worst waste of time. In golf the play is usually so slow that no demand is made by the body for increased air, and the nineteenth hole is always waiting. Besides, the game requires all the strategy and concentration that the player so often requires relief from. Of course, if he is playing golf in order to have an opportunity to out-general his opponent, then he is making a business and not exercise out of the game, and we are considering it as an exercise.

Swimming is probably the best form of exercise for people in general, but again a warning. This does not include fancy diving. Many injuries are sustained in learning to dive, and since there is nothing of importance to be gained from such an accomplishment, the price is too great. Tennis is too fast and too exhausting for any but those who gradually train themselves to withstand its demands, and if this is done, all the warnings hereinbefore mentioned are void. The man in good condition can play even the "nineteenth hole" or try any stunt without damage, because he now falls within the "elastic limit." The same reasoning holds true in all competitive games.

For the great majority of people, some routine exercise that can be done in the bedroom is the most practical, and for this, self-resisting exercises, of which scores are already found to be systematized and detailed, are recommended. But breathing requires special mention because it is usually incorrectly taught.

Stand up barefooted against a wall, heels touching each other and the wall, with as much of your spine in contact with the wall as you can. You will find that in the neck and the small of the back are two normal curves, and if they are not exaggerated, you can just comfortably lay your own open hand flat against the wall between it and your body when the entire balance of the spine is touching. If more room than this is present, there is some distortion, your posture is wrong, and you can better it by trying to straighten up. Be careful in this effort *not to raise the shoulders.* Keep them down and flat against the wall. When you have done this, note the pull on the abdomen and elsewhere, and when you can keep your body in this position, you will have no use for belts, braces, or any other help.

Stay as you are, walk away from the wall, and take a long, slow breath. Take more and more. Take every bit that you can squeeze into your lungs. Hold it a little and slowly exhale it. Repeat, and repeat again. If things turn black or you get dizzy, do not be alarmed. Quit for the day and try again tomorrow. You will find that the same symptoms do not develop so soon. Do not raise the shoulders. Do not indulge in any breathing exercise that calls for raising the arms above the shoulder height, and better yet, do not raise the arms at all.

Muscular development will be obtained from exercise in exact proportion as it is done regularly and purposefully. Weight lifters develop muscle rapidly because they must put *all* their drive into lifting that weight. You can do this in self-resisting movements without the slightest danger of strain, an important matter not safeguarded in weight lifting or working with any apparatus. Light but very fast movements, as in shadow boxing, accomplish an even better result if it is general condition you want, and here "shadow boxing" fills the bill beautifully. Do this for five minutes and do it fast. If at the end of that time you are not puffing hard, you are in condition to stand a pretty heavy fall or sudden emergency.

Before closing this chapter we wish to refer to the tobacco habit just enough to say that, since the tremendous increase in cigarette consumption, a vastly greater number of people are *inhaling* tobacco smoke, and this is deadly. Leaving out of the present discussion all consideration of the destructive effect of nicotine and other well-known poisons generated by the burning cigarette, there is still left what seems to us the worst of the lot, the fact that the blood is unable to discharge its carbon dioxide or to absorb oxygen in an air cell filled with air that is already loaded with the products of combustion. It is probably true that instead of this normal interchange there occurs a still greater concentration in the blood of products that are poisonous to the body than were present when the blood came to the lung to be purified. It is also probable that the average amount of air inhaled with the smoke is so small that the concentration of poisonous gases is greater in the air cell of the lung than it is in the blood corpuscle that came there to discharge its toxins.

Now, if it is understood that carbon dioxide is found in an unstable solution as carbonic acid with an acid reaction, that this is the only outlet the body has for acids which does not subtract from the alkaline reserve by demanding neutralization, and that the amount of acid which is so handled by the normal body in twenty-four hours is enormous, then in the light of our teaching that fatigue and disease are synonymous, it will be seen how extremely important this matter becomes. It is so important, in fact, that we believe a man can do everything else herein advised and never get well if he continues to inhale large quantities of smoke or otherwise fouled air. It has been accepted by some authorities that the solid waste eliminated by way of the lungs in a normal body is approximately equal in weight to that eliminated from the same body through the bowels in the same time.

The reason why the average person who spends a weekend in unaccustomed activity is sore, stiff, and half sick for several days thereafter is that he has used muscles not trained or conditioned for such use, and the abilities of the body to break down this excess sarcolactic acid into harmless forms for elimination are lost to some degree. Then when you make a sudden and unusual call upon your muscles, as in such a weekend, some degree of acidosis results, and it is not until your body has corrected this that you commence to feel normal again.

Rest and sleep are the most certain and the most rapid agencies we have for this correction, always presuming that there is no underlying fault, such as muscles under constant contraction and resulting fatigue. Controlled exercise by increased oxidation assists in destroying acidosis, thereby minimizing the effect of distortions.

Distortions corrected – guarantees rest.

Rest is the only Cure.

CHAPTER XII...EMERGENCIES

While the statement stands true that any pain can be instantly stopped upon proper and successful application of the technic herein taught, injuries demanding immediate and positive control arise more and more frequently as life moves in faster and faster tempo. We would not stand by and watch a man bleed to death or fiddle around trying to find just the exact contact in such a case, even though we knew that, given time, a coagulum would form and no surgical interference would be required. We would first stop the vital losses, then remove the excess load, the strain, and then see to it that rest was secured.

In addition, results from old injuries that have left behind uncorrected distortions do sometimes produce conditions that demand energetic and immediate palliative methods. Suppose you attempt to correct such a condition as cardiac asthma while not yet sufficiently skilled and are unable to locate the correct contact with the patient in the standing position. You have him lie down, which is most difficult for a patient with such a condition, and in his attempt to cooperate with you, he becomes exhausted and cyanotic while you are searching for the exact contact that will immediately clear the condition. You would be unnecessarily hazarding the life of the patient to allow the condition to go that far and should immediately resort to a sedative, preferably a hypodermic, and await a more favorable opportunity before continuing your work.

Nor would we fail to use all active methods if we were called in on a case of coma resulting from uremic poisoning, so long as the life was in imminent danger. Having rendered the danger of death less immediate, we would make all speed to find the contact and correct the condition. Years ago when Dr. Hurley was implicitly believing all the so-called Philosophy of Chiropractic and getting people well by "adjustments," he was making regular calls on a lady of sixty odd years and was making some progress with the case. He says, "She was emaciated, suffering severe intestinal and generative organ troubles and had one of the feeblest and most erratic hearts I ever noted. She suffered excruciating headaches and facial neuralgia.

"I was called immediately upon my return from a short vacation and found that several hours previously terrific pain had developed in the abdomen. Upon examination I made a diagnosis of intestinal intussusception, immediately explained the gravity of the condition, and advised calling in consultation a surgeon and finding out first hand what the chances of a successful operation were as regards the life of the patient. This was done. The family selected a doctor who had before been their physician and was a surgeon of good reputation. His examination and diagnosis confirmed mine, but his prognosis was even more hopeless than mine, and the family decided to leave the case in my hands.

"In such a condition, the result is death or improvement with an extreme limit of forty-eight hours, so we had not long to wait. I used every method I knew at that time to secure sufficient relaxation to deliver an effective chiropractic adjustment; the surgeon administered hypodermics; everyone, including the patient, did all in his power to secure some favorable change, but without result.

"I hesitate to set down in cold type what followed, but it is so important a matter that in spite of arousing a degree of unbelief that may discount the important facts in this book, it is necessary because it is true. The patient died while I was at the bedside. The surgeon and the sister of the patient agreed that all was over. I then immediately took the patient out of bed, more as a last straw than with any hope, stretched the now limp form in position with the help of the surgeon, and gave an adjustment which was so severe that I had wanted to give previously but could not bring myself to it while she still lived, and I had the satisfaction of knowing I had accomplished what had before been impossible.

"We replaced the patient in bed and watched life return. A very fair degree of recovery, with no more distresses and difficulties than had previously been experienced, was made. Thirteen years later (1931) I had the pleasure of meeting this patient again and find that she is now rosy and plump, though just a few months previous she had buried her sister after nursing her for over a year. There is no reason to doubt that she will spend many more pleasant years."

In all of these cases, the saving of *minutes* may mean the saving of life, and this work is too potent, its misapplication is too dangerous, to permit us to take any chances. We require plenty of time, we must not hurry or be hurried, and if an adjustment[4] is attempted under such conditions, our concern for the patient is sure to hurry us whether we are conscious of it or not. Therefore, postpone the adjustment if there is any active method available that can be relied upon, and if you are not entirely familiar with such method yourself, do not take any chances with that, but get the most skilled in its use who is available, and do it at once.

---

[4] The terms *adjust* and *adjustment* were used in the original books. As explained in the Appendix, these terms were later changed to *aline* and *alinement* (spelling purposeful to differentiate from *align* and *alignment*) to avoid confusion with the chiropractic use of the terms.

This book and the instructions contained in it must be concerned with the special subject thereof and cannot go into the indications and contraindications of the therapeutical methods, since that is a whole library in itself. Besides, it would be impossible. The authors of this work do not claim to have more than a rudimentary knowledge of these methods, having found them unnecessary.

The above is meant only to *indicate the point* at which assistance should be sought and not in any sense the conditions in which it may become necessary. Every person who familiarizes himself with the material in this book will have sufficient knowledge of any situation to know when his own work has become ineffective, when it is likely to be, and certainly to know when any situation is beyond his control. If the only thought in your mind is the welfare of the patient, as it must be if you are honest and worthy, the only mistake you can make will be to call help *too soon*, and this mistake is the easiest mistake in the world to forgive; especially is it easy for the patient who makes a speedier and more comfortable recovery thereby.

And now again, and while admitting that these subjects still demand further research, we assert that the technic herein taught is the best, surest, and safest means of securing relief from pain and an uneventful recovery, even in these cases.

Always remember – Rest is the only Cure.

CHAPTER XIII...GENERAL OBSERVATIONS

As was indicated previously in Chapter I, there is a predatory group of political medics whose activities are well worth a few pages in this book, because they are decidedly serving a selfish purpose rather than the public interest which they so blatantly claim to serve and because this book is written for those swarming millions unnecessarily suffering untold agony, who have need of help which the program of the American Medical Association is designed to deny until these millions become so ill they are hospital inmates. They seek to accomplish by law what they fail to earn by merit. Not even satisfied with that, they seek what actually amounts to control of the government, and their program for obtaining this control is so menacing and so well under way and has already accomplished such a large measure of success that a Congressional investigation has been demanded and important support has been exerted to bring it about. The American Medical Association is allied for the furthering of its purposes with similar organizations throughout the world. In every part of the world, the end is the same, that is, the complete control of the individual from before birth until after death. To do this, enormous sums of government money have been used and will be required, and even if no direct abuses appear, the association provides its members with no end of positions in public service much more lucrative than the private practice of the same member would be, and in return he is far more valuable from a political standpoint than he would be otherwise.

The program referred to was first brought to my attention by a booklet published by Dr. B.J. Palmer and entitled *An Invisible Government*, copies of which are undoubtedly obtainable by anyone interested. That program seeks also to influence and control so many other organizations that we can here merely indicate them as including the Red Cross, Visiting Nurses' Association, Parent-Teacher Association, service clubs, speakers bureaus, news associations, pictures, comics, etc. And their attempted and already effective control of insurance companies, labor and compensation boards, health boards, etc., is too well known to require lengthy discussion. Hospitals are so completely under their control, as are all state sanitariums, asylums, and prisons, that no doctor of any sort is, as a rule, permitted to practice therein unless he belongs to the particular clique attached thereto, even though he offers his service gratis.

As early as 1903, the medical doctors who are members of the American Medical Association decided, after lengthy discussion, that there were at that time too many doctors in America and soon adopted a program designed to correct this condition. This scheme divided itself into three distinct activities, namely: first, to obtain complete control of all medical schools so as to destroy some, favor others, and generally reduce the medical enrollment, thus slowing down the production of new doctors; second, to originate legislation designed to create a multitude of jobs, federal and state, for doctors, thus providing places for the excess already in existence; third, to destroy all "irregulars."

The first section was accomplished by means of classifying all medical colleges as A, B, C, or D and making the prerequisites for classification the amount of money available per student per semester in the school. If a school failed to have a certain minimum sum of money to spend per student, that school was not a class A school, and as it was printed in the proceedings of the meeting, the idea was "so that none but rich men's sons might qualify," for a medical education necessarily became much more expensive, especially since all but class A schools were marked for extinction or the courses in these schools were extended along special lines. This has been done, and with a few exceptions, only class A schools are operating today. The newspapers, the only means the public had of knowing what was going on, carried notices to the effect that for better instruction and greater efficiency, "X Medical School" would from and after such and such a date be combined with "Y Medical School," and nearly everybody was satisfied because they did not ask the embarrassing question as to whether the facilities at "Y School" had been proportionately expanded to care for the larger number of students. As a rule they had not, thus decreasing the production of new doctors. Literally hundreds of medical colleges were put out of business by this means, and if the equipment for general practice of the fewer graduates had been improved, some excuse could be offered, but that was not the case. The idea is not so much to produce competent doctors as it is to perpetuate a certain type of so-called scientific medicine by producing "Specialists."

The second section hinged about the adoption in each state of a "Model Bill," governing the relations between the doctor and the public and securing federal legislation which would serve to interlock all of this, supplying the strength necessary to overcome the changes which were necessarily expected, as between one state and another in the final law.

The federal legislation was the first to attract general attention, and the Owen Bill, which would have provided a Department of Public Health with its secretary, a cabinet officer, and the appropriation of $16,000,000 for "organization expense" in the first year, without even an estimate of succeeding years or other expenses, was defeated, but only by strenuous effort.

The situation as it stood at that time may be further clarified by quoting from a lecture given by Dr. Hurley in 1916:

Friends, in order to understand rightly the Owen Bill, it is necessary to know something of the conditions that led up to the framing, so that we must start with the report of the Carnegie Foundation for the Advancement of Teaching, as it refers to medical education. It shows, among other interesting things, that there are 568 persons to every doctor in the United States, as compared with 2000 persons to every one in "overdoctored Germany," and that in many towns of less than 200 inhabitants there are two or more physicians.

Thus, in Burlington, Vermont, there are sixty physicians to a population of less than 21,000, or one for every 333 persons. Nor can this be explained by the assertion that the large towns and cities naturally draw too large a proportion of the doctors, for at Post Mills, with only 105 persons, there are two physicians, and at Plainfield, with 341 persons, there are three physicians. These are merely instances, and the figures can be duplicated in any state. They are cited merely to illustrate the fact that there are now too many doctors. It may be interesting to note that in this state (Pennsylvania) there are 636 people to every doctor, and instead of lessening the present proportion, the medical schools are at present turning out graduates for practice two or three times as fast as the country can assimilate them, making all due allowance for deaths, growth, and so forth.

These figures refer to medical doctors alone and take no note of the number of so-called irregular practitioners nor the number of people who regularly patronize them. There are now in the United States 33,300 of these "irregulars," and 17,813,000 people seek their services in preference to those of the medical school. Eli G. Jones, M.D., of Burlington, New Jersey, states that one-third of the people of the United States prefer someone of the schools of drugless healing.

To increase the earning power of the medical doctor by the raising of fees is impractical, so that the following treatment has been decided upon. First, to reduce their own numbers, deaths, retirement, etc., will help. Second, to decrease the number of medical schools and to make the cost of medical education so high that only rich men's sons can afford it. Third, to destroy all "irregular schools" and to put their practitioners out of business, and last but by no means least, to pass the Owen Bill, which will provide jobs for the balance. To take these points up for consideration in their regular order – the operation of the first needs no explanation. To understand the second, it is necessary to know something of the American Medical Association. It is composed of only 30,000 medical physicians, of which 95% are allopaths. Because it is active politically as well as legitimately and because there is no other organization within the medical ranks, the Association dominates the medical field and every State Board of Medical Examiners. The Association is the power that defines preliminary training, the power that says what shall be the course of study. If any school falls short of the requirements laid down, the graduates of that school are not admitted to examination before the licensing board, which leads to the right to practice. For example, when graduates from three of Chicago's leading schools were refused examinations that would have allowed them to practice in New York State and were given such an obscure reason, the dean of one of the schools said, "Admission of doctors to New York State is more involved in politics than one would imagine."

Another example of the complete manner in which the A.M.A. dominates the legitimate field is the treatment accorded the famous Lorenz, who, after coming to this country from Europe to treat Lolita Armour, receiving $50,000 for his successful work after all others in America had failed, and having expressed his willingness to demonstrate his work publicly, was arrested and fined, persecuted, and prosecuted until he left the country in disgust. And the charge against him was *"practicing medicine without a license."* The trouble was that he did not ask the A.M.A. if he might.

The practical operation of the second remedy is shown by the fact that where ten years ago there were in the United States 186 medical colleges with 26,000 students in attendance and producing 5,400 graduates annually, there are now but 101 schools with 16,600 students and with 2,650 graduates annually, a reduction of about 50% all the way through, and these 101 schools must furnish a course of study that means the expenditure of at least $1000 per term per student. It requires a large endowment as well as large tuition charges to support this, and the weaker schools already have succumbed.

A recent example was the Medico-Chirugical in Philadelphia, absorbed, according to the newspapers, by the University of Pennsylvania for the benefit of both schools, but really put out of business by the A.M.A.

The third remedy, that of the destruction of all drugless schools, will follow in the same way. Every drugless practitioner works under one of three conditions. In Pennsylvania we have an exemption clause in the Medical Bill, granting the right to practice after sufficient examination, just the same as most other states where there is no provision made, and every license is issued by the State Board of Examiners, who are under the domination of the A.M.A., which association has the power of changing the preliminary requirements almost any time. These licenses may all be revoked by the power that grants them for any breach of ethics. Ethics is a vague and elastic word, and may be construed to mean almost anything, so that the licenses of those practicing now are always unsafe.

In many states, drugless people practice without license, and when arrested for practicing MEDICINE without licenses, take the consequences; a few fortunate states have provision for State Examining Boards of Drugless Schools. This is the only legislation whereby the drugless people are independent of the A.M.A., and then not altogether, for the Association continually tries to pass amendments to the law that will restore to them their lost power.

And now we come to the fourth, the Owen Bill. I have shown you the need of some sort to protect the pocketbooks of the regular physician. I can produce in print, confirmation of every statement I have made, so that when I show you to what extent the Association may go under the bill if it becomes a law, I want you to believe that these are the very things that will happen, and I want each of you to ask yourselves how badly you want that bill to pass, and if you do not want it, how are you going to prevent it. I assure you it is a matter of immediate importance.

Senate Bill Number 1 was introduced on the seventh of December, 1915, by Senator Robert L. Owen and has been called the Owen Bill for that reason. It has been referred to the Committee on Public Health and National Quarantine, and the expectation is that it will be passed at this present session of Congress. I have a copy of the bill here, but I consider it unnecessary to read it. I will undertake to obtain copies of it for any sufficiently interested to ask for them. It provides for a National

Bureau whose Secretary shall be a cabinet officer, and although twice before defeated through the activity of the National League for Medical Freedom, the A.M.A. is more determined than ever to pass it, and at the present session of Congress, if possible.

The attitude of the Association is defined by the statement of Dr. John A. Witherspoon, at a recent meeting of the Association in Minneapolis. He said, "The American Medical Association will never rest until there sits side by side with the Secretaries of War, Agriculture, Treasury and other great national departments in the Cabinet of the President, a Secretary of Health for the United States of America." Since then, we can take it as granted that the Association will make every effort to pass this bill, and because it is necessary to oppose its passage, I want to call your attention to the provisions of the bill and the arguments the provisions call up.

The first, and to me the most important, is embraced in the remark of Benjamin Rush, himself a physician, and one of the signers of the Declaration of Independence, that "The Constitution of the United States of America should make special provision for medical freedom as well as for religious freedom. To restrict the art of healing to one class and deny equal privileges to others will constitute the bastille of Medical Science. All such laws are un-American and despotic. They are fragments of Monarchy and have no place in a Republic."

This whole bill is designed to strengthen the hold of the A.M.A. on the whole art of healing, and the Association is composed, as I pointed out, almost entirely of allopathic physicians. The bill specifically states that there shall be no discrimination between schools, but every other similar measure that has ever passed has had a similar clause, and yet since the first report of the Marine Hospital embracing physicians in government service in

1872, not one physician except allopaths is found. There has not been any homeopath, nor any osteopath, nor any eclectic, nor any other but allopaths that have found means to appropriate to themselves any of these berths.

Again, the legislation is entirely unnecessary. The present Public Health Service has more power than any similar organization in the world and publishes more printed matter than the similar services in England, France, and Germany combined. It has demonstrated its competence to handle emergencies by its summary activity in yellow fever and in cholera, both of which diseases have been practically stamped out, and let me remind you this was accomplished not with serums and vaccines, but with sanitary measures and quarantine.

This power has been abused. For instance, the bubonic plague scare in San Francisco, California. This service is not permitted to enter any sovereign state except on the invitation of "proper authority." But the proper authority is not defined, and during the plague scare, although the governor of California demanded the recall of this service, he was unsuccessful. The Owen Bill has just the same kind of limitation. Dr. Walter Wyman, who was head of the service at the time of the plague scare and who was responsible for many of the acts done, at last admitted that "It is a matter of mutual congratulations that NO CASES of plague have been found during this work." Yet he had quarantined the state of California, thereby advertising to the world that there *was* plague there. Dr. White, who had charge of the cleaning of Chinatown, estimated that it would require thirty *tons* of sulphur to do the fumigating, while the state organization did the work in a manner satisfactory to him with only three hundred *pounds* of it.

The power of the service has been greatly enlarged since that time, 1901, but even then, the regulations made and enforced against the will of the state executive meant millions of dollars' loss to the people of the state. The whole story of the scare may be read, taken from official correspondence in the December issue of the *Twentieth Century Magazine* for 1910. This bill adds infinitely more power.

Next, medical science today is not any more a science than it was 400 years ago. It is true that there is more accuracy in measures, and medicines are compounded more uniformly, but many of the drugs in use today are discarded tomorrow and it is the same with their methods. If it were a science, the treatment of typhoid fever could not change from the heroic methods of our own recollection to the sane and successful nondrug methods in use today. Nor could they change from what they are today to the serum treatment now in vogue. The mere fact of the constant changes is sufficient evidence that the medical men themselves are not satisfied with the results they obtain, and I contend that, as long as this condition prevails, the United States government has no right to force me to accept treatment under them, which everyone knows is far from 100%, and yet this is exactly what will happen if the bill passes.

Not the least concern is, according to the statement of Professor Irving Fischer, chairman of the Committee of 100, that "It is a subject which once started will surely expand within a decade, so that millions upon millions of government money will be put into this most needed form of National Defense." No true American objects to spending government money for any necessary thing, but to spend it for a health service which only 30,000 out of a total 140,000 physicians want, and which practically the whole American public decidedly do not want at all, is an outrage. The whole cause for asking this legislation is the plea that it will lower the death rate. That is the platform on which practically all such laws are asked.

Let us look at the results obtained in Connecticut, where the Board of Health has police power and where so-called health measures are carried out in detail. S.B. Munn, M.D., of Waterbury, says that, before the organization of the State Board of Health, the death rate from 1848 to 1877 inclusive (excepting 1852, when no report was published) was 15.66 per thousand. And that from 1878 to 1908 inclusive it was 16.93 per thousand, an increase of 1.27 per thousand after the organization was created to reduce the death rate. And this in spite of the betterment that must be expected under the good sanitary conditions that were obtained. Consider a moment. The death rate was increased 1.27 per thousand in thirty-one years of Health Board activity, where officers were clothed with police power. They entered homes where they were not wanted, they forced all manner of vaccines and serums on people that were well, to keep them from getting sick, so they said.

Besides, this bill particularly empowers the President to transfer to the Health Bureau any other department of the government, excepting only the medical departments of the Army and Navy. When Senator Owen was asked why these were exempted, he replied that, "It would probably be impossible to pass the bill with the hostile opposition of these who are connected with the medical service of the Army and Navy." We wonder why if it is such a good thing for the people, it is not equally good for these. Congress has already refused to consolidate the health services we already have into a single bureau, thus the reason for the clause in the bill. The President may. We are afraid that this bureau, once formed, will become the most powerful of the government departments.

And now we come to things that are possible and that certainly will be done once the power to do them is granted. All the arguments already advanced are based on material carried in the wording of the bill itself, but when the bill is considered in the light of the facts that led up to its framing, the power granted takes on a sinister aspect. The things that we expect will not be done harshly, there is too much money spent already and too much brain work done to hazard the fruits in rash and unpopular measures, so that the first thing to do is to get the public ready for the move that will be made. There was a committee appointed to discover ways and means of accomplishing this, and I quote from their report. "From the experience of past years in state and national efforts to secure favorable legislation, it has been found necessary, if it is to be successful, to precede it with an educational campaign. For many years, magazines, newspapers, and other means of influencing public sentiment have been monopolized by commercial interests. The medical profession has been far too negligent in this particular. Public education must precede legislation."

They started at once this education. From headquarters in Chicago, at regular intervals are sent out to newspapers all over the country – health talks. You can scarcely pick up a paper without running into them. The papers use this stuff as filler. They get nothing for printing it and pay nothing for it. Have you ever read it? Have you noticed that the answer to every question that really requires an answer is to see your physician? Have you noticed that all the old and well-known remedies are, from time to time, declared to be of no value? In short, have you noticed that the whole trend is to encourage faith in your doctor, to encourage more frequent visits to him, and to introduce to your notice the wonderful things accomplished by their serums? I am convinced that one of the first innovations will be the factory inspection of employees. This would provide work for thousands of doctors, and only people without any considerable initiative would be affected.

We already have it in a mild form. A factory inspector enters a building and takes a few cultures. He must find someone to fire, else his services are not necessary. He selects some inoffensive individual who surely has no means of defense, and he must quit. No one cares where he goes nor what becomes of him. If you take a walk in our poorer districts you will surely find an example now, and I have said this is a mild form. What is the result after this is common? It means that the public must build more homes of all kinds, and employ more doctors to run them, and then hustle around and find more people to fill them and so on in a never-ending chain.

I believe the compulsory examination of all school children will be next, and we already have that in a mild form. In New York and Chicago it is not so mild. In New York the law requires their examination in the absence of all clothing and calls particularly for examination of sexual organs, etc. No one knows the reason. Then will come school teachers. The Denver Post contained a dispatch on December 6th last year (1915), stating that school teachers of Atlanta threatened to strike if a regulation requiring their physical examination in the absence of clothing was enforced. The order was so worded that a certificate from the family physician would *not be accepted*. They carried the point, but it shows how the wind blows.

Next will be compulsory treatment. You may think not, but the thing has been boldly recommended, both in New York and in Chicago. And this treatment will be allopathic treatment, as all the examinations will be allopathic, for no other doctor will find any chance to enter this service, especially if he is not a member of the A.M.A. And all this means more hospitals, more doctors, and more expense. Is it hard to see where the millions and millions of government money will go?

In Wisconsin this year, twenty-four adults, normal physically but slightly unbalanced mentally, were sterilized before their *release, as cured.* Is that compulsory treatment? What happened to the personal liberty and the pursuit of happiness our constitution warrants to every individual? Where did all the cry about eugenics come from? These people had committed no crime and there was no assurance that their offspring could not be as healthy as the average, physically and mentally.

Remember the necessity of reducing the ratio of doctor to population and turning potential patients into active ones. If it was scientific, even then it would limit personal liberty in an unwarranted degree. Since it is absolutely *not* scientific treatment they recommend, and since Dr. Cabot, one of the foremost of American physicians, admits that he correctly diagnosed only 53% of the cases that came to autopsy in ten years' time, how are we to be sure that even the treatment they used will be indicated by their school for the disease that is really present? You simply cannot be sure of anything except the inspections and some kind of treatment. Do you want to be one of those active patients?

Bear in mind, please, that I have directed my remarks at the A.M.A. and not at the stay-at-home family physician. There are many, many upright, honorable men in the medical profession. They may be mistaken, as any of us may be, but no one could conceive them as political job hunters. Medical freedom is the thing that we demand, that every American should demand, as did Benjamin Rush, and it is a subject that is worth your earnest consideration right now, for this bill will pass unless there is considerably more adverse agitation than has already developed.

At the next session of Congress it appeared again, was again defeated, and for the third time as Senate Bill Number 1, went down to a third defeat. The World War intervened. Mr. Harding expressed himself as opposed to the Owen Bill, but after election it was discovered that he was in favor of the France Bill, one introduced by Senator France of Maryland, a medical doctor, member of the American Medical Association and a close personal friend of President Harding. More trouble was experienced with this bill because in the interim a number of changes had been made in it, the most important of which was that the name had been changed to "A Department of Public Welfare" and the statement was made that public welfare embraced every rightful activity of government, therefore every department of the government should be subsidiary to this one and the A.M.A. would control it. It was at length defeated.

The next was the Budget and the inclusion within it of the Brown Bill, our old acquaintance in slightly different dress. This bill became federal law. This federal law, according to the statements of its sponsors, the A.M.A., gives all the powers sought. It enables that group of politico-doctors to absolutely dominate your daily life and the lives of all your near ones. It has been clearly stated that such powers will not be used or attempted until the time is propitious, because any sudden interference with the personal liberties thereby abrogated would prove a boomerang, but if the field is carefully watched, little by little the thing can be done.

The first state to pass the "Model Bill" and put into effect its provisions was Indiana. And there are, as a result, more than 16,000 medical doctors on the public payroll in that state, or one doctor supported by every 200 people. So we see how the second division of the program operates. The ultimate intention is by controlling all hospitals, asylums, homes, etc., and all industrial and mercantile establishments and by establishing "Group Medicine," now coming so largely into vogue, to make the general practitioner not only unnecessary but to see that there is nothing left for him to do. Thus we see the objective in the change of character in the instruction offered to new medical students.

If section two is completely accomplished or nearing that point, an order can be easily made, such as has been declared to be the objective, "To close every doctor's office in America," to force anyone who is sick to report at a certain allocated hospital where they will receive, willingly or unwillingly, whatever procedure the doctors in group practice there think advisable, and to pay a price for such, irregardless of results or value received, which will be determined by reference to the income tax files. Such methods once and for all dispose of every irregular osteopath, chiropractor, those skilled in the present method, or what not. In order to accomplish this, a tremendous number of new hospitals and similar institutions will be required, and means for acquiring them at public expense is embodied in the legislation already in force and still sought. It is menacing, destructive, and probably a self-destructive program, because it is built upon and gathers strength around a group of claims as to efficiency, which are false.

CHAPTER XIV...FURTHER OBSERVATIONS

The Spanish built the Panama Canal.
The French built the Panama Canal.
De Lessups built the Panama Canal.
The Americans built the Panama Canal.
Major Goethals built the Panama Canal.
The American Medical Association built the Panama Canal.
Roosevelt built the Panama Canal.
Engineers built the Panama Canal.
Common labor built the Panama Canal.
The Oregon Short Line built the Panama Canal.
The Southern Pacific built the Panama Canal.

Each of the above statements, with the exception of ten and eleven, will attract supporters. Each supporter will advance what seems to him good reasons why no other statement concerning the above is true. Even in the case of ten and eleven, the obstacles they threw in the way of the program, the profits they were deriving from the absence of the canal, were strong arguments for its construction, and so some may even agree that ten or eleven is true, and the more ignorant of the facts concerning the development of this great work the supporter of any of the above statements happens to be, the more certain and radical he becomes that the statement he supports is the only true one.

This is the danger we are all subject to in stating any case. No one can know all the facts about any large matter. It is physically impossible, and we understand this too well to allow the impression to find lodgment in the mind of the reader that we are bound to be or possibly are capable of being entirely conversant with all facts in any case, the case of the A.M.A., for instance. We try to state the facts as truly as is possible in what follows and throughout this entire book.

In relation to the Panama Canal: The Spaniards had the visions and dreamed the dreams that centuries later became the Panama Canal. A charter for this work was issued and preliminary surveys were made about 1541.

Without the work of the French and De Lessups, it might have appeared a hopeless task, even to the American people. Without the American people and government, and as long as the Monroe Doctrine remained in force, the canal probably would not have been completed. Without Major Goethals, the A.M.A., and the unlimited resources of such kinds as then were known, the canal would have taken such a toll of men and material that it could not have been carried through against the public opinion that would surely have developed.

Without Roosevelt, who acted in direct opposition to the reports of his own appointees – engineers of the highest standing, it would have been a sea-level proposition and possibly not yet in satisfactory operation. Without America's own type of engineers, the thing would have been impossible to build and still impossible to operate, because the "electric mules" that form an essential operating unit, to mention only one, were an unheard-of proposition at that time.

Some of these factors, of course, are more important than others, and the control of fever, partly made possible by the A.M.A., was extremely important. It is said that, figuratively speaking, there is a dead man under every tie of the old Panama Railroad, yet fever control has made the zone a safe and healthful place in which to live. But the trouble with the

A.M.A. is that they take *all* the credit for this work, leaving none to the important Sanitary Engineers, who having other work to do and no ulterior motives, are thus not articulate. And the A.M.A. gets away with their misleading propaganda that it was entirely *their* work, experience, and knowledge that brought this great work to a successful completion.

So it is with *all* of the propaganda, including statistics they so consistently publish. For instance, they claim to have lengthened the span of life. That is true in a sense, but it is not important really, as already noted on pages 82 and 83, when properly understood. Out of 1000 people, the average age at death is not more different than is to be expected from other causes to be noticed than it was ten, twenty, or fifty years ago. Modern surgical and therapeutical methods are saving for a few brief and painful years a large number of subnormal newly born. If they live longer, they usually become public charges and sources of constant expense, either by imprisonment or disease, for years before they finally pass on. So far, little progress has been made in the reduction of these too numerous subnormal newborns.

The actual increase in the average span of life, if any, is due to better housing, better clothing, better food, better sanitation, and less onerous labor. They claim to have reduced the death rate from diphtheria to one-third of the previous percentages. From one angle this is true, but from another angle it is *not* true. If the figures are seen in their *true* sense, it is found that out of 1000 people, just as many die of diphtheria as before the use of toxin or antitoxin came into vogue. Before the introduction of the toxin antitoxin, no case *was* diphtheria until and unless it showed the characteristic throat of that disease, almost always deadly. While now everything is diphtheria when a swab of the bad throat shows Klebs-Loeffler bacilli.

For instance, an acquaintance of the authors, never under any but medical care, frequently suffered from sore throat. A few days following the usual big Thanksgiving dinner, she had a recurrence of the trouble, so severe that she called in the family physician. The medical doctor, after taking a swab, pronounced the presence of diphtheria on the one side of the throat and quinsey on the other side. That is getting it down to a fine point, we think. Of course, she got well in a week or two, as no cast formed, and another case of successfully treated diphtheria was recorded. The family was quarantined the required time.

True, under the serum treatment the vast majority of such cases get well as they always did when they were called by other names. The only deadly sort, the kind that produces the cast on the throat and tonsils, is just as deadly now. The lower death rate is obtained by adding this tremendous number of spontaneously recoverable cases to those previously diagnosed as diphtheria, calling them all by that name and then stating that out of 1000 cases only one-third as many die.

It is doubtful if the serum method is any more effective than the older methods, or at least if it is sufficiently better to warrant the grave risks that are taken by all who submit to its use, for every time it is used on a healthy patient that person is in serious jeopardy. For instance, it was announced over the radio a short time ago that a doctor, having a fresh supply of serum and wishing to use it, inoculated about forty-two healthy school children, sixteen of whom died thereafter with diphtheria. The reason was given that he had accidentally given diphtheria toxin instead of diphtheria toxin antitoxin. This is most difficult for even the gullible to believe, for what use does any practitioner have of diphtheria toxin in his office, and if the mistake was made by the pharmaceutical company, why did he not place the blame on them? However, the report was immediately hushed up, the public was unable to get any particulars, and of course, the doctor went free, although guilty of at least manslaughter. It is demonstrated consistently that when the medical doctors receive a fresh supply of serum and try it out on a large group of school children at one time, the hospitals are unable to take care of all the resulting cases of illness.

Vaccination is another matter upon which all sorts of false propaganda are constantly being put out. The worst epidemics of smallpox in the history of the modern world occurred in Germany and Japan after compulsory and universal vaccination had been enforced. It is true, we have very little trouble with smallpox today in America, but again, the sanitary engineer does not get his proper credit, for smallpox is essentially a filth disease and we are no longer filthy in civilized countries and especially in America.

Epidemic control after floods and other calamities is another opportunity for propaganda, but the control of food supply and water supply and the concentration of refugees in places where shelter, warmth, and rest are supplied have probably very much the major importance, and let us here state that some of our best sanitary engineers in this specialized branch are also medical doctors and members of the A.M.A. A great work, an immensely valuable work, is being done by members of that organization, but they have overstepped the bounds of public service *as an organization*, and have prostituted their great power to selfish interest. They themselves know better than any other can how far they are from a basis sufficiently productive and accurate in the healing of sick people to rightfully *force* their own methods upon unwilling subjects. And by pursuing such activities, they divorce themselves from the confidence and respect of thinking people.

If vaccination protects, the protected ones need have no fear of the unprotected. If diphtheria toxin antitoxin is a sure protection, there is no need for quarantine, and so on. *Reductio ad absurdum.*

Now since the above is true, there must be a powerful reason back of it. Some powerful force must be constantly exercised to maintain such a condition and make the constantly increasing inroads on private liberties, and there is.

That force is representative of the most powerful groups of America, and besides the drug manufacturers and serum producers, the Standard Oil Co. and others have such tremendous facilities for the production of drugs, especially the coal-tar products, and such a capacity for profits from them that they could give away all their other crude oil derivatives and still remain in business. The serum manufacturers have a somewhat different proposition. They must continually foist upon an unsuspecting public products that are advertised especially in insidious ways as possessing wonderful powers, even though they change their products overnight without bothering to change their advertising.

The life insurance companies must have a basis upon which to make rates. These are the actuarial tables. They are made up from mortality tables, "expectancy of life" is derived, and the rates are thus set. Medical doctors necessarily obtain high position, usually on the Boards of Directors, and some companies use vast sums of the premiums paid for the advertising and propaganda thus originated.

The movies in particular are loaded with this advertising in forms the spectator seldom traces to its true source or meaning. When you see on the screen an osteopath, chiropractor, or any of the drugless healers made ridiculous, or a medical doctor aggrandized, you can be reasonably sure there was money talking in that picture. Hack writers, cartoonists, and even more serious authors have fallen under the influence to such an extent that you scarcely can pick up any printed thing without somewhere coming into contact with some phase of this untruthful propaganda. Watch for it, and from now on you will be amazed at its frequency, its cleverness, and its real power.

The public schools, the universities, *every public* institution, every conceivable direction, and every conceivable means are used to maximum effectiveness, and all is directed by the best brains, the most highly developed technical skill, and supported by the greatest money powers in America. No wonder it is dangerous.

No one could object to any legislation the A.M.A. cared to ask for as long as it confines itself to government of its own affairs. There can be no good reason for denying a governing group the power to govern itself, but when that request for power oversteps this limit and has a destructive effect upon the public in general or upon any competitor, then it falls within the definition of class legislation and opposed to the fundamental principle of American Government. It is class legislation the A.M.A. seeks. Nearly every bill presented to any legislative body by any group is in some sense class legislation, and that should be sufficient reason to deny the bill, for no matter what it reads, no matter if the reader sees what is sought to accomplish or not, the mere fact that some special group wants such a bill is sufficient evidence that the group in question sees a method whereby to dispose of some obstacle and seeks to profit at someone else's expense, usually the expense of the general public in the last analysis.

By this criterion, the only legislation the A.M.A. is entitled to, whatever the political division or subdivision, is a law which limits the scope of its activities. That is the only sort of law the osteopaths, the chiropractors, the Aquarian-Age healers, the plumbers or farmers, etc., are entitled to. Under a legal and judicial system that theoretically guarantees equal right to all and special privilege to none, there can be no other answer.

It is very certain that no group having accomplished special privileges, as has the A.M.A., is going to voluntarily relinquish them, and therefore the first duty in a legislative sense of all non-drug or anti-drug groups, including the advocates of Aquarian-Age Healing, should work to secure the passage of the following or something similar.

LIMITING DEFINITION OF THE PRACTICE OF MEDICINE

The practice of internal medicine shall be defined as that procedure which introduces into the living human body, through any natural or artificial orifice, any substance known or believed to have therapeutic value, as distinguished from nutritive value, for the cure or prevention of disease in that individual.

The practice of surgery and all other specialized practices shall be separately and likewise defined.

For instance, Aquarian-Age Healing should be defined as a science, art, and philosophy for the removal of strain and the correction of distortion in the human body. As applied to the individual human body, its fundamental principles are based upon the identification of fatigue as disease and the only cause of pain. Over-stretched or contractured muscles are muscles in a constant state of fatigue and muscles in which rest or restoration cannot be obtained, and a condition in which thereby pain, fatigue, and disease constantly accumulate. This accumulation of fatigue and its poisons is marked and measured by the degree of acidosis, hydrogen-ion concentration, present at any moment, generally or in a localized area, and furnishes an exact measure of the approach toward death of the patient or the part, at that instant, since death is exhaustion and exhaustion is the iso-electric point of the body colloids. These muscular conditions result only from distortion. Distortion results only from strains which have exceeded the elastic limit of the body that sustained them at the moment of their imposition and are represented by structural disrelationships which can be measured by determining departures of the body that sustained them from its normal gravity line.

Since in any structure, distortion of the whole reaches its greatest magnitude at the center of gravity of that structure, any distortion of the human body reaches its greatest magnitude at the center of gravity of that body. Since in any structure, in order to restore it to normal relationships it is necessary to restore its center of gravity to its normal position, so in the human body this is the only requirement for the correction of any distortion or disease, because without distortion there is no disease.

Aquarian-Age Healing, based upon these principles, teaches the correct measurement of these distortions, the correct estimates of the approach to death, and a simple, easy, totally painless, complete, and permanent method for the restoration of the center of gravity of the body and all its parts to their proper relationships, thereby destroying distortion, removing strain, stopping pain, correcting acidosis and all its attendant evils, and completely restoring the body in all its parts and as a whole to perfect health and function.

It has been amply demonstrated by experiment that living tissue, free from strain and accumulation of waste products and when properly nourished and under proper temperature conditions, is immortal and that, moreover, it will destroy disease within itself and gradually restore itself to normal condition in the process of its own cell division. Since proper food and temperature conditions are easily obtainable by everyone, since rest and the removal of waste products are the only other essentials necessary for the immortality of the cell, since this Aquarian-Age Healing provides rest and the removal of waste products of the cell, and since the human body is merely an organized system of cells constantly undergoing the changes that make them perfect and immortal, immortality of the body with restoration and preservation in the maximum degree of all the powers of the body, including the mind, is the end sought and taught herein as ultimately possible.

In its wider conception, Aquarian-Age Healing applies the same rules to all human relationships.

The fundamental idea in such a program is that it specifically limits each group to adherence to and the practice of the principles thus specifically defined by these limiting definitions. Anyone wishing to practice under one or more of these groups would be under the necessity of qualifying under each, a condition not now realized, because at present most members of some groups and a few members of certain groups step beyond their own boundaries without any qualifications and form a grave danger to their public. These limiting definitions guarantee to the public the true qualifications possessed by the practitioner of any method or methods and, in addition, create for the first time an open competitive field where each system stands or falls on its own merit, and the public will be guaranteed of honest goods and service.

This would limit each man to the practice he professes, thus forcing each system to stand or fall of its own intrinsic worth or lack of it. For instance, the allopath doctor could no longer practice electro-therapy without properly preparing himself and securing the necessary certificate. Nor could any other practitioner, regardless of what he represents himself to be, pursue the practice of or make use in his practice of anything not included in the limiting definition set down.

This solution is so simple and so eminently fair that even the medical doctors themselves must assist in its realization or be marked as sympathetic with the A.M.A. program for the elimination of competition. To withhold assistance in this matter means that they believe that most people are fools, incapable of knowing when they are feeling badly or better, or else that they do not care how they feel, thus allowing them to go along merrily with their program into a future of power, peace, and prosperity.

Copy this, have your neighbors do the same, sign them, and either send them to the authors in care of the publishing company of this book, or hand them to the doctor to whom you entrust your life. If he is in sympathy with the ideals of liberty upon which government should rest and upon which permanent government must rest, and wishes for the development of the best and the suppression of the worst by the only fair court –

the public – he will help build the local conditions necessary to its realization and join himself with this publication in the international movement to put it into activity.[5]

The undersigned will lend such moral aid as is possible in his own legislative district, whenever and as often as may be necessary, in the effort to write limiting definitions for each and every branch of the Healing Art.

Signed_____

The undersigned, in addition to the above, pledges all his influence, be it great or small, in the effort to have his own personal doctor join in this movement.

Signed_____

---

[5] This request is no longer in effect.

CHAPTER XV...SAFETY FIRST

At the beginning of this book, reference was made to the prophecies concerning the Aquarian Age. It will be remembered that one of the conditions identifying the Aquarian Age and one of the requirements to fit anyone for participation in the benefits, the joys, the comforts, and the happiness which are to separately mark this age from all others is honesty in the hearts of men. That can only mean that a man with dishonesty in his heart has not brought himself into harmony with the requirements of the Aquarian Age and therefore is a destructive factor and a man to be avoided in every way by those who are sincere and honest.

Those who practice this healing art as a means of livelihood or as a means of furthering, in the greatest degree, the happiness of those with whom they come in contact, have above all things else the requirement of absolute and unswerving honesty if they are to merit your slightest confidence, because when you put your health in their hands, you are giving them care of your most precious possession. A man may lose anything else and start again, but having lost his health, whether through incompetence, ignorance, dishonesty, or carelessness of his own or of the doctor he consults, his ability to start again is always impaired and all too frequently destroyed.

A statement is often repeated in this book that the information herein conveyed will, by its proper application, permit any intelligent person to restore to normal health anyone near and dear to him. But conditions often arise when it is desirable to have the assistance of one whose business it is to care for the ill. If you are convinced of the truth of the teachings contained herein, then with the help of this chapter you will be entirely capable of making the proper choice of a doctor.

The authors of this book, the originators of this work, in an effort to provide satisfactory assistance of this sort have been engaged for many months in the training by personal instruction of individuals they believe to be especially qualified, and every person so trained and qualified has received a diploma, a facsimile of which is here shown, and bearing on its face a clear statement of the abilities developed. Please note that the least grading which we consider satisfactory for service to the public is 85% and that the grade actually attained is shown upon the same diploma. The system of grading is such that no personalities of any sort may enter, and at this writing (1931) no student has complained of his grading. The same methods, without any change, will be followed in all future teaching unless means should be found to insure still more accurate and impersonal grading.

When and if you go into any doctor's office, regardless of what he pretends to practice or what he calls himself, and if he uses the methods detailed in this book or falling under the definition of this work as given in Chapter XIV, you should see prominently displayed in that office that diploma. Look at it; note the grading upon it; see if that man has prepared himself for professional work. And if you do not see the diploma at all, ask that doctor how he qualified himself, where his diploma is; insist upon seeing it, and if it is not shown, be certain that he belongs to one of two groups, namely and first, that he has been a member of a class for professional instruction and failed to make a passing grade and also has refused to take advantage of opportunities that were extended to better that grade, when naturally he would not show his diploma; or second, that he is attempting to make use of this work in a professional way without having properly qualified himself therefore, because, of course, it is true that both time and money must be expended by anyone who wishes to acquire the training necessary thereto, and there are those in the healing art as elsewhere who will not make the necessary effort, but will attempt to secure rights and privileges, confidence and respect equivalent to that properly belonging to those who do.

Any diploma lost, destroyed, or stolen will be instantly replaced upon notification to the proper sources, so there can be no excuse of this sort offered, and as a result, the absence of such a diploma in the office of anyone attempting to do this work professionally is prima facie evidence that that man is dishonest, is unqualified, is not worthy of your respect or your confidence, and for the good of your health is to be avoided at all costs.

He may have bought in the open market, just the same as you did, a copy of this book, and he may be attempting to use its teachings. But do not be deceived. Any man who has previously been engaged in any branch of the healing art other than this has so many things to unlearn, because these teachings are so diametrically opposed to all that have gone before, that he is not more competent but actually less so than you yourself to make a practical application of these teachings, as we have amply proven in our class work by the greater difficulty of teaching this section to professionals of any school than we have experienced in teaching the same work to any layman.

AQUARIAN-AGE HEALING

DEVELOPERS

Hurley and Sanders

Founders

THIS DIPLOMA CERTIFIES THAT

HAS COMPLETED THE STANDARD COURSE IN AQUARIAN-AGE HEALING
ON

IT WAS PART OF THE UNDERSTANDING UNDER WHICH THIS
COURSE WAS TAUGHT, THAT NO STUDENT COULD BE RECOMMENDED
BY THE UNDERSIGNED TO THE PUBLIC AS SUFFICIENTLY SKILLFUL TO
MERIT THEIR CONFIDENCE WITH A LOWER GRADE, MATHEMATICALLY
ARRIVED AT, THAN 85%   THIS STUDENT ATTAINED
A GRADE OF   PERCENT.

IN WITNESS WHERE OF WE HAVE HEREUNTO SET OUR HANDS
AND SEAL THIS   DAY OF

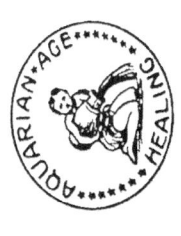
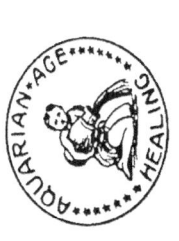

AQUARIAN·AGE HEALING

In order to prepare properly for professional work, it is necessary to master, in addition to the teachings of this volume, all that theoretical knowledge and technical skill which we have organized as section two and section three. That work is written as Book Two of Aquarian-Age Healing [Bio-Engineering] and is legitimately obtainable only by students who have graduated in our professional classes.

This limitation is made for two reasons. First, because the dangers warned against in this book are so greatly multiplied in the advanced work that it is unsafe for anyone, no matter how well educated or skillful in other methods, including the medical doctor as well as others, to attempt their use without personal instruction and close supervision during the class work. For this reason, our classes are limited to twelve students under any one instructor at any one time. Even with this close supervision, we have never yet succeeded in running a professional class without some slight accident occurring.[6]

Second, because so much work, requiring a considerable expenditure of money, remains to be done in the development and perfection of these methods and since in the very nature of the thing, endowments cannot reasonably be expected, the authors of this work must provide those funds from their own earnings, so they are endeavoring to run classes only at a profit in order that these profits may in turn be used to advance the work. For that reason, all material is copyrighted, all rights reserved and otherwise protected from any use by unauthorized people, and the professional who attempts to engage in the work without having entered one of our classes is therefore cheating us, besides doing great damage to you.

But the occasional dishonest person who has entered our classes and has then given the work at second hand without the proper authorization, equipment, or class routine, is not only a cheat but a menace to the public as well, because he is neither

---

[6] Dr. Hurley's further research into the 1940s changed this perspective, virtually eliminating risks in application due to minimizing forces used.

competent as a teacher nor prepared to put in the time required nor the effort necessary to convey that instruction properly. Since it is only through proper channels that our diplomas are issued, the possession of our diploma with its passing grade is your protection as well as ours against dishonest people.

It has been a serious problem with us whether even this Book One should be put on sale in an unrestricted way, because of the dangers that are inherent in the work and that cannot be separated from the enormous healing potential that is present and that makes this work of so much greater value than anything previously known to mankind.

We were influenced to take that action and finally decided upon it on account of several factors. First, the exorbitant charges of worthless, or at best comparatively inefficient, assistance to the sick. Second, by the fact that there are vast numbers of people who cannot obtain any assistance at all. Third, personal teaching and training of professionals in this work has progressed to the point where it is possible to put on lay-class instruction at very reasonable charges and, upon request, in any district where this book is placed on sale. Desiring further information concerning this, fill out the attached blank and forward to the publishers.

It is earnestly recommended by the authors, if any difficulty is experienced in the application of this teaching, that you take this action, for we repeat again what we have said repeatedly throughout the book: this Section One,[7] as taught herein, positively will restore any person who is sick to full and normal health, regardless of age or condition, when it is properly applied, and its proper application can be successfully taught in this class work to any layman without previous instruction or knowledge of any sort beyond the will to learn and the

---

[7] *Section One* refers to *Bio-Mechanics*. Aquarian-Age Healing originally was divided into four sections. Sections Two, Three, and Four comprise the advanced material of *Book Two* and are referred to as *Bio-Engineering*.

ability to understand his own language. And this statement rests on trial and proof that is as positive and definite as every other statement contained within these covers.

There is slowly forming, as a result of our teachings and the spread of this knowledge, an international organization that we call the "Layman Healers League." Every reader of this book who finds some value in any phase of the things set down is invited to join this league. In its present embryonic form, no great promises are made as to what it will do nor what it will mean, but we believe that sufficient indications have been given of its possibilities and its enormous potential value to mankind. There are no dues; there are no obligations.

If in the future any dues should be imposed, they will be determined entirely by whatever local group you yourself belong to with full knowledge as to its purposes and its responsibilities. It is our hope when this work is a little further advanced to maintain regular communication, through the printed page and the local organizations, with every member thereof and in that manner acquaint each one with the results of further research and development that has practical value. There are many other activities more or less closely allied in nature with the broad purpose of this work that will be included as rapidly as they develop after such becomes possible.

Some of the immediate, practical, and personal values to be had from such a league will automatically develop just by knowing who else in your immediate vicinity is interested in the same work, in the assistance you can be to each other by virtue of talking over amongst yourselves the problems and difficulties of adjustment and the course of events under adjustment that you each are experiencing. And by doing work in common for each other in a group, the true meaning and the proper application of the methods herein taught will become clear much more rapidly than by any other practical means, with the exception of organized class work. Besides, no one can be sure how valuable such a connection would be in case some sudden emergency arises. It is a great help to have someone to confer with if a really serious illness suddenly demands attention.

The proper understanding of medical encroachments upon your personal liberties under the guise of Public Welfare and the methods in use to rob you of those liberties will very rapidly appear in an occasional meeting, concerted action can be taken for the preservation of those liberties and even if that resulted in nothing more than the protection of your children from the definitely proven bad results of vaccinations and inoculations, it would by that means alone have many times repaid you for any time and energy used in such a league.

But there is another element of inestimable, immediate, and continuing value in such a league. Through all the history of the healing arts, from the earliest down to and including the last, there have been and are individuals who find their own particular method of the greatest value in some particular disease. And because these same people are unable to obtain the proper results by this same method in another group of diseases, they rapidly come to the point where they will insist that they are making the best use of their particular method by not applying it in the second group, in spite of the fact that some other practitioner is successfully using the same method in the second group and not in the first.

It is to be expected, if you get good results in the application of the method herein taught in a case of hernia or varicose veins that may first have demanded your attention, that you will believe the method is good for that, but you might have your doubts as to its value in a case of scarlet fever or gonorrhea. But if you are a member of such a league, there would certainly be someone in that league who had tried it and found it equally effective in these or any condition that you might unexpectedly be called upon to care for.

In closing we wish to announce that it is our intention at the first opportunity to establish a headquarters for direct mail inquiries from such league which will receive due consideration and proper and rapid reply, for it is our earnest desire to make this book and the message it brings of permanent and increasing value to you.

CHAPTER XVI...INTRODUCTION TO TECHNIC–DYNAMITE

This book is dynamite. No one with any common sense would get rough with dynamite. If he needed it, he would take care to understand how to make it do the things he wanted done without getting himself into trouble with it or blown up by it. The same is true of this book. It will teach all that anyone needs to know in order to completely master all pain and disease. But if ignorant, incompetent, or careless application is made of the material contained herein, the writers must not be held responsible for bad results any more than the dynamite maker should be if someone blows himself up.

This is no cry of wolf. The wolf is actually about. Both of the authors have themselves suffered much pain and distress due to wrong results that were sustained in the early development of the principles herein written – and in spite of every care that could be used to prevent just that. It was the correction of such disturbances and their analyses that to some extent led to the final development of the true facts.

In case bad results are experienced, do not get excited. Make up your mind that you did something wrong. Take your time, be absolutely sure you are right *this* time, then go ahead. If you are right *now*, your troubles will be over *at once*. But do not permit a wrong condition to continue. It may get worse and worse. It may take on the characteristics of acute disease. It may lead to fatal result, and if you are unable to fix what you started to fix, get help that is dependable, preferably a doctor who knows and uses the material herein contained, and tell him all about it, show him as nearly as you can what you did and why, and everything will be all right. There is only this to remember. Nothing but our teachings is necessary to get anybody well who is sick, no matter how he became ill or how long he may have been sick, if only he will stay alive until you can do the work necessary, which is only a matter of minutes to one skilled.[8]

The contents of this book are not opinions or theories except as specifically stated in each case. There is nothing else but fact, demonstrable at any time, any place, and by any person who will sufficiently study the contents to prepare himself properly to make his test of any value. Every result claimed as obtainable is as certainly obtainable by a proper application of the principles of this work as the sum of four is obtainable by the proper application of the principles of arithmetic. And also it is just as impossible to get any other result in the one case as in the other. This can also be stated as follows – that when the expected result is not obtained, there can be no other reason for it than an improper application of the principles. This work is exact, specific, scientific, and inflexible.

No one has any right to any opinion as to the value or lack of it in the material herein presented until and after he has sufficiently mastered the principles involved and otherwise qualified himself to make a thorough test of said contents. If such a test is made under these conditions, no other result than that promised can be had. By the above we mean, as has been explained, that this Aquarian-Age Healing is not only a new method, but based upon entirely new conceptions, and no M.D., D.O., D.C., or any other kind of doctor has any basis for

---

[8] See Foreword regarding cautions, considerations, and contraindications.

opinion without forming such by careful study and application of the present material.

As early as 1915, certain startling recoveries occurred as a result of chiropractic adjustments in Dr. Hurley's office. The first was a case of pulmonary tuberculosis. After months of unsuccessful treatment, this young man was taken out of a state sanitarium by his father when he was notified that the son could not live through the night. Someone persuaded the father to have Dr. Hurley look the case over, and when he saw the patient, he was of the same opinion as the sanitarium authorities. However, thinking the patient might be made somewhat easier and after explaining the possibility of immediate death under an attempted adjustment due to the fact that hemorrhage began upon the slightest movement and everyone being agreeable, Dr. Hurley proceeded. He had an immediate "hunch" that something of vast benefit had occurred after the adjustment, as the result was so instant, continuous, and beneficial. A complete recovery was had in the course of the next year, and all during that time, although this patient was under constant observation, he never was adjusted again. The plain fact was that Dr. Hurley feared to make another, thinking it might spoil what was evidently so good. He takes no credit for this recovery, frankly confessing that to this day he is ignorant of just exactly what he did that night that produced such remarkable results or just how it was done. He tried on numerous occasions to repeat, and frequently with some degree of success, but never with the startling and instant change that was then secured.

Later, a man with a very bad case of asthma was his patient. One slight adjustment completely stopped the attack. He was not seen for months, then another attack, another adjustment, and it was all cleared. He had been having constant trouble before the first adjustment, none between the first and second, and none for months afterwards. One Christmas Day when the turkey was on the table, he came to Dr. Hurley with another very bad attack. The same adjustment, the same exact work, and no response at all. The dinner spoiled. What was left of the turkey after the guests had finished was hung outside, and the cats ate it while he worked on the asthma. No result. Several weeks of work. A consultation was called. No result. The man was taken by Dr. Hurley to a chiropractor in a neighboring town, where some slight improvement was secured. When almost home again, the car hit a bump in the road and instantly the asthma was worse than ever. Arriving home, Dr. Hurley gave him the exact adjustment he first had given, and instantly the trouble was all gone with no return. And that was fifteen years ago.

Again, a man came complaining of lumbago, and an adjustment was given by Dr. Hurley. He had instant results and arose from the table with no pain left. He had a very large inguinal hernia (rupture), completely descended when he came in, and had been so afflicted for years. The next day and from then on, much to his surprise, there was no sign of it to be discovered except some slight looseness of the ring, which gradually closed up without further attention.

Shortly after, one day a husky fellow working under a car in a nearby garage strained himself in such a way as to cause an inguinal hernia to descend. Dr. Hurley, happening by, noticed him holding his side and asked the trouble. Upon examination he was invited to Dr. Hurley's office, who expected to fix it right up. He worked his heart out on that case, tried everything he knew of – *no results*. In this case he charged the patient nothing for the work because of the complete lack of results.

Another case. At closing hour an old patient brought in a man for attention. As Dr. Hurley had to make a certain appointment by train with only sufficient time to make that connection, there was no time for talk, examination, or anything but the adjustment, given with as much care as was possible and the usual exactness. Record of the adjustment was made on the train, and when the man failed to report as directed, the mutual friend was asked the reason for the delinquency. He replied that the man was cured. "Cured of what?" Dr. Hurley asked, and was then informed that the patient had been stone deaf for many years and had completely recovered his hearing before he left the office. There was no return of the trouble on last report, ten years later.

Other similar cases could be given, but the above are believed to be sufficient to establish the point to be made, which is that a tremendous potential exists in the human body; that when the principle which changes that potential healing force into *available* healing force is correctly understood and used, everyone who uses it thus, *will get well.*

The search for this principle has occupied a large part of Dr. Hurley's time since the incidents related occurred, and within the last few years the solution has gradually appeared. As these years went by and these developments appeared, one thing, which he called "The Great Prescription," formed itself clearly. No one was ever known to get well without its help and many are known who would have died without it, regardless of what other methods had been or were used. It follows.

Good Food
Good Shelter
Plenty of Exercise
Interest in Life
No Excessive Fatigue
Plenty of Rest

Pin it securely in your memory; use it all the time. It will never lose its potency, and among all prescriptions it is the only one the same today as it was 3,000 years ago.

CHAPTER XVII...TECHNIC[9]

As this work is based upon the correction of all distortion (strain), we must know what distortion is. The root of the word itself comes from torque (twist) and means the twisting away from. So in the human body any twisting away from its normal relationships is distortion.

It now becomes necessary to establish the normal of the human body so as to be able to determine the degree and amount of distortion present. As we must have an accurate point to begin with, we place our patient's feet together, heels and toes even, as shown in Figure 7. This serves two purposes, for not only does it give us a starting point and a basis for comparison, but it also reduces the ability of the body to cover up and hide its distortions, for it now has only a small base upon which to balance.

Next, find how the body weight is distributed over the feet. To have perfect balance in the human body without strain, there must be symmetry, so we must establish a normal median line from which we can measure departure from normal or loss of symmetry. This line is established by dropping a string from

---

[9] Much of the information in this chapter was later updated and clarified by Dr. Hurley, though it gives valuable insight into the technic. The changes are outside the scope of this book, and the chapter should be read with this in mind. See Foreword for more information.

the ceiling or doorway and attaching a plumb-bob on the free end about one inch from the floor. This plumb-bob should point to the spot marked A in Figure 7, which lies on line B and corresponds to a point midway between the two heels.

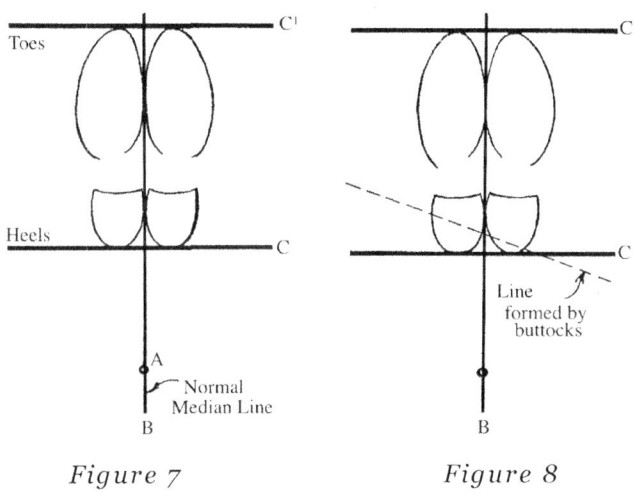

Figure 7   Figure 8

With the patient's feet placed as indicated and the string in its proper place, you must now stand directly back of your patient with your feet on exactly the same median line B and pointed in exactly the same way as your patient's, but at least three feet away from him. Your patient is clothed only in an apron opened all the way down the back and has his shoes on, for you are going to balance his body to the condition under which it is normally subjected, and all standing, walking, and working is done with shoes on. Now have him close his eyes and keep them closed. Tell him to relax every muscle possible in the standing position, and constantly tell him to keep his weight equally distributed between his two legs. This is of utmost importance, for if it is not done, none of your determinations can be depended upon. With his eyes closed he is unable to see the extent he is swinging from his upright posture and will in this way show more nearly his true distortion.

Note and record any departures of that body from its normal median line as indicated by the string. This line should pass from the point midway between the heels, midway between the knees, exactly on the line formed between the thighs and the buttocks, exactly on the entire line formed by the spine in the center of the back and between the shoulders, exactly in the middle of the neck and head. The hips, shoulders, and head should be level, the arms should hang evenly at the sides of the body, and the right and left sides of the pelvis must be alike and must not deviate from the standard set by line C and C[1] of Figure 8.

Now that your patient is standing completely relaxed (or as relaxed as his distortion will allow) with his eyes closed, and you are standing behind him in the proper way, make a drawing and record of what you see, for instance as follows, which is an actual case:

1. Line between thighs right of string.
2. Line between buttocks left of string.
3. High hip right side.
4. Median line in lower back left of string.
5. Line between shoulders left of string.
6. Middle of neck left of string.
7. Head tilted to left side.
8. Low shoulder on left side.
9. Anterior buttock on left side.

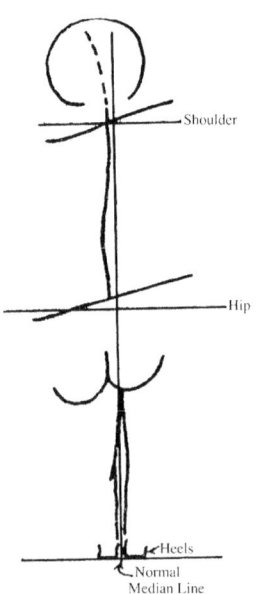

All of these points, beginning with number one to and including number eight, can be seen and recorded while standing a few feet back of the patient. But to determine number nine, it is necessary to step up directly behind your patient and lightly place a stick, ruler, or some straight object so that it barely touches the most prominent parts of both the right and left buttock. Compare this line formed with line C you have marked on the floor as in Figure 7. In the case just recorded the two lines would look as follows in Figure 8. This shows the left buttock is anterior or further forward (that is, further away from you) than the right buttock. This last determination is the most important of all to get accurately, for if you are careless in this one, the damage you will do will be widespread and difficult to correct.

As this section of our work is concerned only with the soft tissue, you must note particularly areas of contracted muscles and make note of any outstanding abnormalities so as to direct you in judging your progress, for contracted muscle cannot rest and lack of rest means accumulated fatigue and disease. You do not need a knowledge of the skeletal framework for this Section One work.

With all these deviations from normal recorded, you are now ready to place a jack (in the form of a contact) under the sagging corner of that body. This is done with one of your fingers, all others keeping clear of the body, and with a pressure no heavier than that which can be comfortably borne on the eyeball. IT MUST NOT BE HEAVIER. It is not PRESSURE that gets the results; it is ACCURACY. We do not PUSH or FORCE the body into its normal relations. That will take place normally and perfectly under a correct contact.

RULES FOR TAKING CONTACT[10]

1. The contact is ALWAYS on the anterior buttock. It has been definitely proven that the buttock may become anterior but not posterior, so we must LIFT that anterior buttock OUT. Therefore, your finger must NEVER have any hint of forward pressure in taking either a standing or bench contact. You must get under the flesh of the buttock and bring that *anterior* buttock BACK TOWARD YOU.

2. The contact is *usually* (but not always) on the side of the erector spinae muscle that is the most contracted in that region as it passes on either side of the spine from the pelvis to the ribs. When both sides of this muscle are heavily contracted, it indicates that the sacrum is very anterior and must be LIFTED "Out of the Hole." It has been definitely proven mechanically and practically that the sacrum can and does slip anteriorly and *cannot* slip posteriorly due to its articular surfaces. Never allow anything to happen to your patient while he is relaxed in any way that will cause the sacrum to move anteriorly or your patient will *always* get worse.

3. In general, it seems that the more a body swings away from the string, the further out on the anterior buttock is the contact. If the departure of the body from its normal median line is slight, the contact generally falls on the anterior buttock near the center of the body. See Figure 9.

---

[10] Superseded by Dr. Hurley's later revisions. See Note in Appendix.

4. We never adjust anything but the sacrum.[11]

5. We never adjust any sacrum except from the INFERIOR, the force passing slightly superior and mostly posterior.[12]

6. We never take contact on the sacral base, as this would tend to increase distortion.

7. We never adjust directly on the sacrum, but use the soft tissue to correctly influence the sacrum.[13]

8. Place the contact so as to tend to reverse the distortion.

Having made a record of the distortion, you must now determine where the proper point of contact is that will correct that particular distortion. You will note three main types of distortion in Figure 9. The one marked No. 1 is the simpler distortion of the three and more easily corrected because the body has made little adaptation.

But it is tiring to stand that way, so the next thing the body does is to adapt itself more completely, and then you see a body like No. 2, standing more in line with the normal median line,

---

[11] The Appendix changes this to: The effect of the contact is principally through the center of gravity via the sacrum and secondarily on every bone, muscle, and functioning tissue in the body. As the sacrum is the structural center of the body and holds all other parts in correct or incorrect relationships through muscles originating from it, directly or indirectly, we need concern ourselves with the position of the sacrum only. The correct or incorrect position of all other parts of the body, correct or incorrect posture, is an indication of the correct or incorrect position of the sacrum. Any work done on the other parts of the body for the purpose of alining it almost invariably moves this structural center further from normal and, therefore, is detrimental from the standpoint of health.

[12] The Appendix changes this to: We never move any sacrum except from the *inferior* and *anterior*, the direction being slightly superior and mostly posterior.

[13] The Appendix changes this to: We never take contact directly on the sacrum, but use the soft tissue to influence the sacrum correctly. Only the posterior surface of the sacrum is presented to the worker, and no contact on this surface can bring it backwards.

but with muscles tighter and harder. In too many cases, the distortion is so severe that even this adaptation is not sufficient to allow continued movement, so the body makes the last adaptation as shown in No. 3. If the distortion becomes any worse after this, the patient may no longer be able to stand at all, for this is what happened.

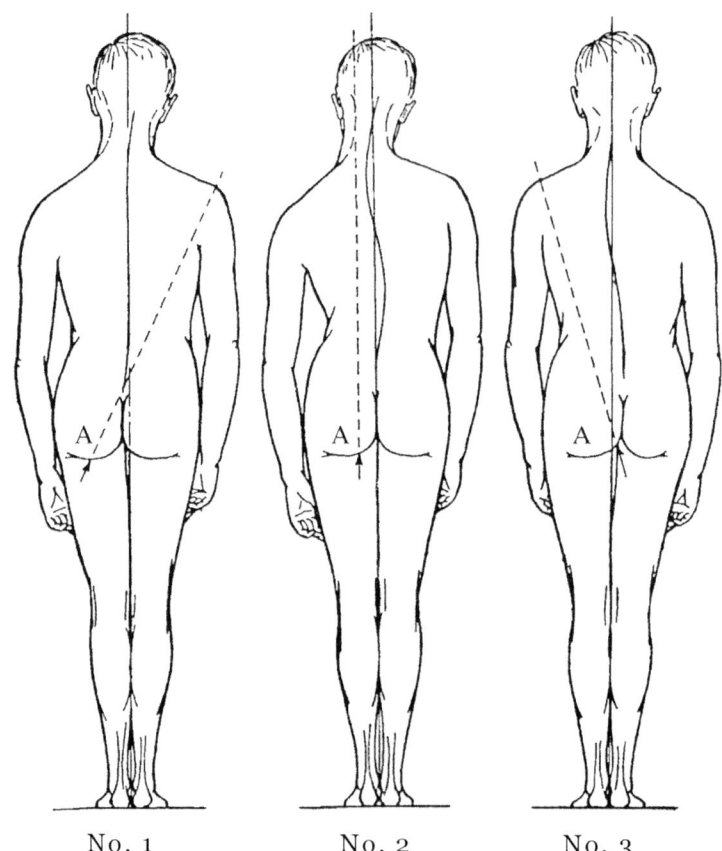

No. 1   No. 2   No. 3

Three main types of distortion showing point of contact and line of drive.

Figure 9

In No. 1, the left buttock is anterior, and the entire body has rotated to the left. But there is a limit, and as the body settles more and more into that weak spot, some adaptation must be made to bring that body back into its center line, so the pelvis is moved over toward the right to minimize the extreme left anteriority. This brings many parts back into the normal median line as shown in No. 2, but at the expense of the musculature, which results in increasing fatigue.

If the distortion continues to get worse, in order to keep that left side from becoming any more anterior, the pelvis is moved further and further to the right, as shown in No. 3. This is necessary to maintain the best balance. If No. 3 becomes any worse, then the upright posture becomes impossible for that body, because the last possible adaptation has been made.

The greater the vitality of the patient and the stronger the musculature, then the greater is the adaptive ability of that body to the distortion present.

Now that you have satisfactorily determined the anterior buttock and having in mind that you must bring that anterior buttock back to you with your contact as well as restore or maintain the proper relations of the body to the normal median line, and having determined what type of distortion is present and where the point of contact is to be and the approximate line of force, take contact as shown in Figure 10. Before you touch the body, note the point of greatest deviation in that body from normal. This frequently is at the juncture of the neck and shoulders.

When you lightly take contact, notice if that point of most noticeable distortion becomes better or worse. If it becomes worse, take your contact off IMMEDIATELY, make a recheck, and determine what is wrong. You must instruct your patient to report any changes felt the moment they are felt. Never hold any contact if any bad report is given. This point cannot be too strongly stressed. You will produce either good or bad results with your contact and they will occur NOW and not later. That is one of the satisfying things about this work. You know while you are working whether you are getting results or not and whether they are good or bad. You do not have to wait.

Your criterion is – decrease in distortion means relaxation and rest. Increase of distortion means contraction and dis-ease.

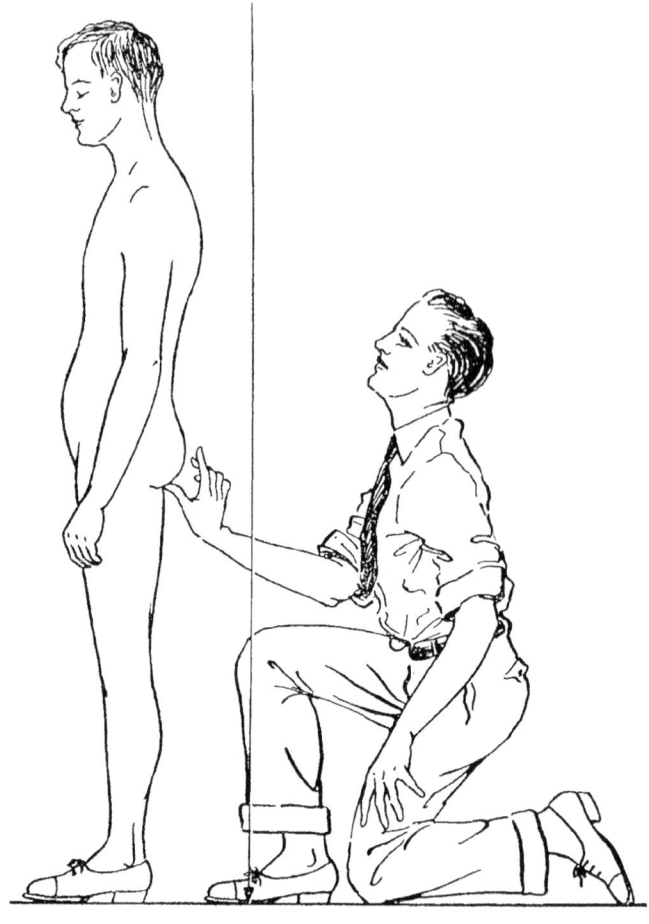

Figure 10

If you do not heed this warning and insist on holding a contact that is wrong, your patient will fall over and he will be sick. If there is no one near who is skilled in this work, it may be necessary to call in someone to give a hypodermic to produce temporary relaxation of muscles you caused to contract due to the strain you placed on him by your wrong contact. Of course, it is more desirable and to the best interest of your patient to call in someone skilled in this work to undo the damage you caused, for otherwise the damage will be to some degree permanent. It is possible to produce a typical case of appendicitis in three minutes in certain types of distortion, and it will continue to grow worse and will endanger the life of the patient if something is not done about it. Again, the only correction is the removal of the actual damage done, and as the disturbance was produced by mechanical means, so the correction must be made by mechanical means.

When you get that contact under the right spot and in the right direction, the low shoulder will raise up, the head will lose its tilt and will come up, the hips will become level, the rotation of the pelvis will be gone, the patient will report lessened or the total disappearance of all pain and discomfort and will feel rested and relaxed. You will soon learn to note all curvatures, both side to side (scoliosis) and front to back (lordosis and kyphosis).

When all these evidences of distortion are relieved or gone, then mark the spot you are holding with a skin pencil or crayon, and make also a line to indicate the direction of force you were using. Of course, you cannot mark this direction exactly as you were holding it, for sometimes it scarcely enters the body at all but is coming almost directly back toward you, but you can indicate it sufficiently to know yourself what it means.

Some might feel as though the use of the string is a bit of a nuisance, and wonder why it is necessary. The importance of this item will be fully realized the moment the reader stops to consider the fact that it is the distortion of the body as a whole that makes it become diseased, and if distortion of only a part is taken into consideration, then the diagnosis is very incomplete and entirely undependable. The entire distortion must be diagnosed and must be corrected as a whole, and any operator who objects to the use of the string or some similar device is not interested in getting his patient well, for this is the *only accurate way* of diagnosing distortions, and if distortions are not correctly diagnosed, how then can they be intelligently corrected? This is very carefully taught in our class work because of its prime importance. It is the *one* criterion that will always truthfully report your work as good or bad – without fail. It is only bluffers who are afraid to face the issue who will refuse to stand a patient behind the string afterwards, as well as before working on them, and thus put their work to a test.

Now you are ready to place your patient on a bench, table, or some suitable arrangement. It must be comfortable so that the patient can lie without feeling a need for moving while you are working. Your patient must never move without your permission. If he moves while under contact, it produces an adjustment that is usually wrong and is many times most difficult to correct. The hips must have a roll under them, raising them up, as shown in Figure 11. This position not only lifts the buttocks up so you can get the necessary contact, but also leaves the abdomen free for the testing of any trouble there.

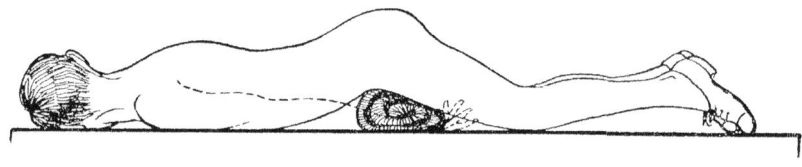

Figure 11

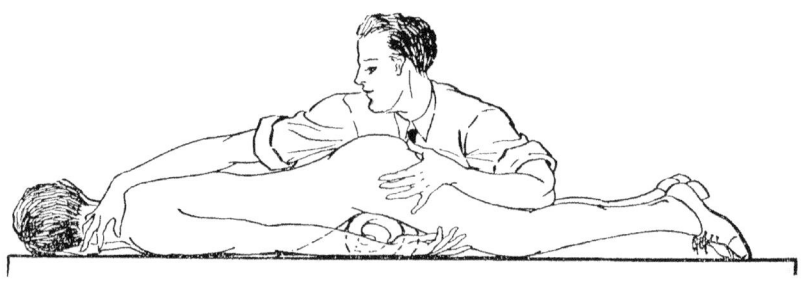

Figure 14

With your patient face down on the table, be sure he is comfortable; then tell him to report every tender place that you touch. You have a skin pencil in one hand, and with the other free hand you use just one finger to test for tender places on the back and legs, as will be indicated, and make a mark with the skin pencil on the *exact* spot reported as tender by the patient. These tender places are areas under strain and you are going to remove the strain.

For a systematic marking of these tender areas, begin at the base of the skull in the median line. Lay your testing finger on the skin at the spot indicated, and with enough pressure to carry the skin and tissue under it along, move your finger back and forth, a stroke about an inch long, about three or four times and *crosswise* of the long line of the body. This is enough pressure to bring out tenderness if it is present. Do not hurt your patient. If he is oversensitive and has many tender places, go very gently. If you hurt him, he will tighten up, and it will make your job many times more difficult.

If that spot tested is reported tender, make a mark; and then take each space between the bony tips that mark the middle line of the back, placing a mark on each one reported as tender, ticklish, or numb. Continue in this way to the bottom of the spine (including the coccyx). Now follow out around the buttock, always rubbing *across* the muscle fibers, as this brings out the tenderness better. Come back to the center of the body by way of the crest of the hip bone; then go over the other buttock in the same way. Now go up to the base of the skull again, this time about two inches to the side of the line previously followed, and go all the way again to the bottom of the spine. Do this on both sides.

The proper *routes* to follow in locating tender areas of the back are shown in Figure 12 by a solid row of dots. You will also see from this figure the proper distance between your test points. If you test areas closer together than those indicated, you only waste time and energy, for the few strokes you were

told to use in locating tenderness is sufficient to cover the area
in between the marks as shown.

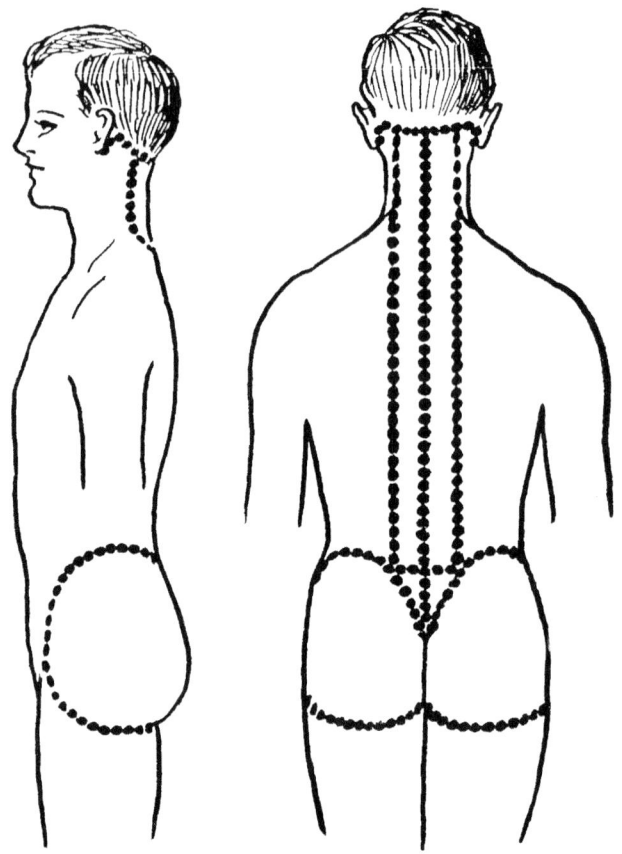

Figure 12

Now carefully feel of your patient's abdomen, not hard
enough to make him contract, but firmly enough that he can
report any trouble. This is the only way any abdominal
palpation should be made, for in this position all the organs
drop towards the table and lie in your hands, and you can gain
a very clear idea of their actual condition. If the patient is on
his back, the organs drop back into the abdominal cavity, and it

is almost impossible to separate one from the other and impossible to palpate some of the deeper organs at all.[14] Just try it, and you will be surprised at the difference. There is no need to mark the tender areas found in the abdomen, for you will not be able to see the marks when you need them, so just keep them in mind.

There are areas all over your patient's body that are tender and you could spend a day marking them up, but we believe we have shown the major places to look, that is, the front and back stays and the diaphragm, as brought out in our chapter Evidences of Distortion. However, if your patient has some particular complaint that does not fall in the areas indicated, then go all over that area, marking the tender spots, and clear all these along with the ones found in the routine marking.

You are now ready to make bench contact. Decide which hand you are going to use for your contact hand and which side of the table you will work from that will afford you the greatest comfort, for you may have to hold that contact for some little time at the first when you are just learning the work and developing skill. Before you do anything with that contact hand, locate the most tender areas on your patient that fall within the areas marked A on Figure 13. Place your free hand upon that spot and keep it there, testing when necessary, until all the tenderness is gone from that spot. This is your starting point in the clearing up of all the tender areas in any body.

With your testing finger ready on that one spot in this area (no other area will do; this is the one right place, for this is the area through which all force must pass from the trunk to the legs and thence to the ground), place the thumb of your contact hand exactly on the mark you made for your contact point when the patient was in the standing position. Keep the remainder of that hand as free as possible from the patient's body, touching only enough to guide your line of force. Never let any part of

---

[14] In practice, the therapist does not palpate individual organs but rather the abdominal musculature.

your contact hand except the thumb touch the buttock. It is permissible to touch the thigh only. Use as nearly as possible the same line of force as you were exerting in the standing position, being especially careful to lift up. To do this, you will find it necessary to keep the contact arm and elbow quite low as shown in Figure 14 [page 174].

This contact on the bench is no heavier than in the standing position. The moment that contact thumb touches the buttock, begin testing that one spot in that one area on which your testing finger is located, and have your patient report each time you test it whether it is "better," "worse," "same," or "gone." Your patient needs no other vocabulary than this while you are working on him, and in this way he directs you so that you can do the work systematically.

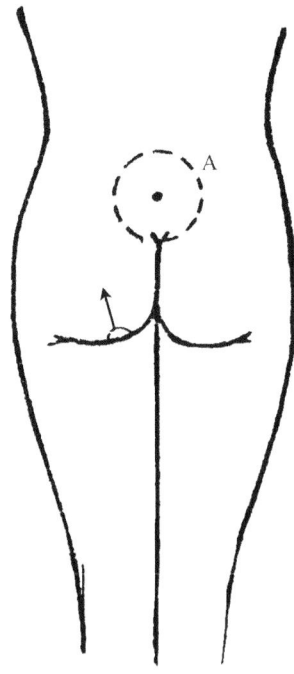

Figure 13

If that spot you are testing is reported "worse" when you first put your contact on, then take that contact off immediately and figure out what you did that was wrong. The probability is that you did not put your contact on properly, that instead of lifting towards the ceiling, you pressed slightly towards the floor in the attempt to gather up the flesh under your thumb. This must not be done. Or perhaps you did not get as near to the direction you marked for your line of force as you should have. Do not get in a hurry. This work must be done carefully, lightly, accurately, and intelligently at all times. Figure it all out; then try again.

When you take the proper contact and that central spot is tender no longer, then, using this as the center of a circle, begin clearing all the tender areas around it, gradually enlarging your circle until all are gone, frequently returning to that first spot to be sure that it remains free from tenderness and that you are still progressing and not sliding back.

There is a very important point that must always be borne in mind. Suppose the point of contact and the line of drive is as shown in Figure 13. You place your contact thumb carefully, lightly, firmly, and steadily on that spot and in the direction indicated, and the spot you are testing (at the lumbo-sacral articulation) is immediately reported better but not gone. Never move that *point* of contact unless you stand your patient up behind the string again, go all over the case, and figure out just why you were wrong last time and why you are right now. The thing to do now is not to move your contact point, but to change your *line of force* very slightly, either to the right or left of the way you are holding it, and you will find out which way is correct by your test. You will realize how slight a change is necessary when you visualize the line of force, as shown in Figure 13, projected to the shoulder. Now if a slight move were made to the right from that point of contact, the force would then be directed to midway between the shoulder and the neck. Another slight move, and the force would be directed to the middle of the neck. Now, your one right point and direction that will correct all distortion in that body *may* lie somewhere in between, so the changes in your line of force must be very slight. Remember also that your contact is affecting the tissues of the body in the head and feet as well as immediately around your point of contact.

Now that you have placed your contact and found that it is good because it reduced the tenderness of that first spot you are testing, you must find whether you have to move your line of force to the right or to the left to entirely clear that spot. If you move it slightly to the right and the spot grows more tender, then you know that direction is not correct, so you return again to the original direction of force and begin to change it slightly to the left. If that clears this one tender spot, then you test until you find another. Then gradually and slowly moving your line of force IN THE SAME WAY, you clear all places marked. Frequently you will find a tender area in the neck that is very stubborn, and in the attempt to get it out, you begin to reverse the direction of your line of force and may clear the neck. This frequently happens unconsciously with beginners, and almost invariably you will find that this neck area is being relieved at the expense of the first areas cleared, for if you go back and test them, you will find that all the tenderness has come back again, and then you know that you are wrong, that you have taken strain off of one area and placed it on another, so you must take that contact off and start all over again in the same systematic way.

When you have finally perfected that contact so that *all* the tender areas of the back are gone, then you gently slide your hand under the abdomen, after cautioning your patient not to move, and you find and remove any remaining tenderness there. If this work has been right and your contact is right, by now your patient will be extremely relaxed and his tissues will shake like jelly, which is the normal condition of relaxed muscle tissue and the only state in which fatigue poisons can be properly and completely removed, and during all this time he is getting increasingly better due to this relaxation.

Now that every spot is clear, stop a moment – think exactly where it is that your line of force is emerging from that body. It may help if you will mentally project that line to the ceiling or wall or some object, and when it is clearly in mind, give a very light thrust directly toward the spot you picked out and just heavy enough to slightly spatter a cranberry. If you were right and your thrust was accurate, you will see the effect of that light thrust all through the patient's body due to its relaxed condition.

Let your patient rest a moment, then begin to test all the areas that were tender when he was marked up, and see if you were so accurate that they are now all gone. If a few have come back, then take that same point of contact and the same line of force you just used, perfect it again so that all tenderness is again gone, and give another light thrust. When you have taken all the tender areas away, then you are through adjusting.

Let your patient rest for half an hour;[15] then have him stand up behind the string and note changes. If your work was properly done and your patient is not suffering some acute ailment, he probably will need no more work done for a week or more. If your work swung the pelvis so that it is now rotated the opposite way and the other buttock is now anterior, it is all right to leave it that way, for the body will gradually balance itself. Do no more work. If after a week this opposite buttock is still anterior and the patient feels better and better, do not touch that person. This mistake is made by many of our students in the beginning until they have had some experience. They will give an adjustment,[16] taking the proper contact on the anterior buttock, and do a good job and swing the patient the other way, and the patient feels wonderful and thinks that a

---

[15] The Appendix updates the requirement for retesting and rest. Neither is necessary during the session.

[16] *Alinement* replaced *adjustment* in Dr. Hurley's terminology in 1936.

miracle has occurred. Then the next day the patient wants some more of it, and the operator wants to do some more, and as the opposite buttock is now anterior, they take contact on the opposite side. Usually it takes only a touch, and the patient will swing right back where he was before any work was done, the body becomes heavily contracted, and the patient becomes very ill right away. The operator soon learns that it is now much more difficult to work on that body due to the heavy contractures produced.

Never change your contact from one buttock to the other except in the following case. Suppose in the case with the left buttock anterior, the adjustment swung the pelvis until the right buttock was anterior and the patient felt no particular relief. When that patient comes again for the second adjustment and the right buttock is still anterior, do not work on him. Wait for at least three days. Then and then only, if the right buttock is still anterior and the patient is not improving, your contact will be on that right buttock. This means that your first analysis was not correct, that the distortion shown by the patient at the time of the first adjustment was not the true distortion but an adaptation to it. If that is true, then you will find that your contact will never again leave that right buttock, for it is the one that is really anterior and your progress will be continuous from then on.

Be exceedingly careful in changing your contact from one buttock to the other, or you will consistently undo all the good you could ever do.

It is frequently the case that in order to clear all tender areas your line of drive has been changed to such an extent that it is going almost directly towards the ceiling, and you feel that it is impossible even to hold that tissue any longer because your thumb is almost ready to slip off and that it would be entirely impossible to drive at all on that contact. Do not be discouraged about this. If you find yourself in this situation, every tender spot is gone and you are almost ready to slip off, get all the speed you can while maintaining that angle, and give your thumb a little flip, which is all that is possible. You will be surprised when you make the check test to find that even this has been really effective. If necessary, repeat and repeat again.

In acute cases or in cases where definite and positive results must be secured, keep right on as long as any tenderness in the back or in the affected area can be found. You need not hesitate to adjust every few minutes, because, in fact, for the best results you must keep plugging away, for the distortion is serious and the contractures heavy or the patient would not be so sick. And by doing this, you will positively control any trouble whatsoever in a few hours.

During this time if you keep your patient warm, there will be a continuous and increasing sense of improvement, and instead of becoming fatigued, your patient will feel stronger and stronger.

But if you have cleared all the tender spots, then give the thrust, and many tender places return, the explanation lies in very inaccurate and careless work or in one of the following complications:

First: You tried to hurry. You cannot hurry.

Second: You were interrupted at a critical moment and did not go again over *all* the spots before you gave the thrust.

Third: You have chosen a point of contact that will rotate the sacrum in the correct direction, but you did not choose the best point and the sacrum is not moving *exactly* right.

Fourth: You may have a compound distortion to deal with. This will be denoted by a crooked line between the buttocks, that is, the line between the buttocks describes an S or ⟩ . If this line is a straight line, no matter in what direction it points or how much rotation of the pelvis it shows, it is a simple distortion and may be corrected by following the above instruction. But if this line has a bend or kink in it, even though it appears to lie in the right place in relation to the string and to be pointing in the right direction, it is a double or compound distortion and very difficult to handle under this Section One; but if care and patience are used, it can always be done. Such cases, however, will make better progress if taken to a recognized practitioner of Aquarian-Age Healing who has been trained to correct all distortions.

Fifth: Your work may have been so good that additional sore spots have developed due to the relaxation of the deeper structures. If you note a great deal of relaxation and the patient agrees with you that this is true, that he feels wonderfully relaxed and strong again, you may call it a day. Or you can work on such a patient all day long with continuing and increasing improvement as long as any distortion shows. But you must check up frequently behind the string if you do this.

Section One technic, as taught in this book, does not warrant any heavier thrust than indicated. Do not take chances. Play safe. The patient's health, comfort, his very life may depend upon your accuracy. You are again cautioned to never make a thrust of any kind until you have eliminated every tender spot. It is much more to the advantage of your patient and yourself to stop after having taken only test points and contacts than it is to give the lightest adjustment if that adjustment is the least bit wrong, because even this preliminary work has produced some degree of result and the change may be favorable, but if you give an adjustment the least bit wrong, the net result will be bad – and may be very bad. Do not adjust at all until you are absolutely sure you are right.

COMMON ERRORS

1. Careless marking of tender spots. If this work was not necessary, it would not be insisted upon. It is absolutely essential. True, in cases unable to answer questions intelligently, only those skilled in the advanced work should be allowed to make or attempt any correction whatsoever. If you do not mark, you save no time, you only waste time and lay up

no end of trouble for yourself and your patient by being careless or trying to hurry with any part of this work and the marking in particular, to say nothing of a lack of good results and almost certain bad results. Do the marking exactly as taught. Any less is insufficient; and more, superfluous.

Nervous, hasty, indecisive, or prodding movements, too heavy or too light pressures, fail to elicit the tender areas. They only make your patient resentful of pain you are causing and nervous and irritable themselves. Or if they are of slow reaction time, you pass from one spot to another so rapidly that they have no time to report. Having carelessly passed one spot or marked it in the wrong place (and your patient is always conscious of this), he immediately makes up his mind that the marking is not so important a matter and ceases to give it his attention, with the result that your marking is incomplete, your test points do not constitute a satisfactory test, and your contact and adjustment are both bound to be wrong. One or two experiences such as result from this may be the only thing that will teach you, but at every point we are trying to save you grief. You may disbelieve if you like; you will suffer the consequences if you do.

2. Too light a test. After you have a contact that is right, the pain is *gone*, and you need not fear to go right into the spot that was sore such a short time before. If you do not have enough confidence in the result of your contact to warrant you in making a deep test, you certainly do not have enough confidence in it to deliver the adjustment that goes so much deeper and is so much more permanent. Your patient has not reasoned all of this out, but senses it just the same.

3. Testing after the adjustment. After the adjustment, remove all contacts from the body before beginning to test to find if any sore spots yet remain. Of course, it required considerable time to establish the contact you just used, so you may have a tendency to hold it while testing, but if it was correct, as it should have been, everything is now finished. If it

was not, then it is not good enough to try again without further test. The main objective is to find out what results were produced by the adjustment, but as long as you hold contact you cannot find out.

It is difficult both for the professional and the layman to understand the dangers of this work, and even at risk of becoming tiresome, we must once again with all our force warn you to follow this technic in every detail. Do not permit any variation at all.

It is reported by one of our patients who was interested in the work, yet knew little concerning it, that one day an employee suddenly was stricken with a "pain in his back" so great that he immediately had to quit work. Our patient took this employee and through his clothing, without any of the preliminary steps, placed a contact and made a thrust, instantly stopping the trouble. The man immediately went back to work and had no further attacks, but such work is so dangerous that neither of the authors of this book would consider it nor undertake it. We know the dangers, and we know what an immense amount of "Luck" we would need to have in order to properly correct any trouble in that way. One thing that might happen in such a case is that the immediate pain might be corrected but the sacrum left in a worse position, one where vital structures would be influenced instead of the big muscles of the back, thereby trading a merely painful condition for a new one that might later threaten life itself.

Everyone knows that anything that is productive of good is capable of producing an equal amount of harm if the process is reversed. So it is with this work. There is in it a terrible potential for good with an equal potential for harm. But if you will carefully follow all that is herein taught, you will remove disease processes by removing their cause, namely slight slippings of the sacrum with the resulting strain placed on the muscles of the body, and your results will be considered as miraculous as compared with past cures that have been experienced in the ordinary run of life. With this knowledge and skill, you will be better able to take care of those dear to you than anyone skilled in any of the past methods. Try it and prove it.

Note: *The Appendix was originally published as a separate booklet in 1936. It was included free of charge with the purchase of books after that date, and it was inserted at the end of Book One in later printings. The Appendix clarifies and updates the technic instructions in the original book. Dr. Hurley continued to research and improve his technics throughout his career and made many important revisions that were never published but were taught in his later classes (especially after 1940). See Foreword for more information.*

APPENDIX

The purpose of this book and appendix is to enable its every reader to obtain freedom from pain and disease for himself and family. Merely to read the book without applying its technic will not accomplish this in any degree whatsoever. You are failing in your whole duty to yourself and your family unless you make the necessary application of the teachings now in your hands. To understand the principles set forth in this book is of some advantage, but the whole intention that led to its writing, publication, and open sale will be completely defeated, so far as you are concerned, unless you now make a personal application of these teachings.

Do not lay the book aside with the impression that Aquarian-Age Healing is merely a fine idea but perhaps not a workable one, and do not fail to use it thinking that perhaps you will need other instruction or further training in order to proceed safely in the development of its values. The whole instruction is here before you. Nothing else whatever is required but your effort. Remember that it took years of study and investigation in order to perfect this work. Now, in order to secure the benefits of this work you only need to apply its teachings. The authors will be very glad to hear from you as to the outcome of your efforts.

The technic herein taught is easily learned without other training. It is intensely practicable and highly efficient. During a period of some years now, many persons have used this text as a workbook and without any further instruction have restored others to health.

Continuous and critical experience with any matter clarifies the thought as well as the technic of that particular subject. This has occurred with Aquarian-Age Healing. In 1934, there was issued free to all purchasers of record of *Book One* at that time and to all purchasers thereof since that time, a certain bulletin, the contents of which are now embraced in this appendix. This bulletin was issued to clarify certain points in technic and in line with the intention of the authors to be of continuous service. Since it has proved to be of real value and the opportunity is presented by the exhaustion of the original supply of bound books, the bulletin is now included in the appendix without change in price of the book.

The principles of Aquarian-Age Healing are entirely new. The method of healing presented is not only unique but simple and scientific. All methods of the past employed in the healing art have each established a certain standard of results. Now it is found that the results with which people once were satisfied under old methods of treatment are by comparison with those of this new method very poor, most unsatisfactory, and entirely unreliable. With the introduction of these new principles, science is added to art and betterment is continued to cure. It is known now that man may and should attain a far higher level of health and efficiency than he has ever believed possible.

If you will read this book, then study it for the sake of acquiring additional and valuable knowledge, not viewing it as a piece of *literature*, you will find it possible, nay highly desirable, to treasure this work as one of your most valuable possessions, even to the point where you will be seeing to it that your friends have like opportunity to acquire the knowledge and help.

The book, even without this appendix, has amply demonstrated by its wide sale and use, not only the accuracy of the teaching, the efficiency of the work, and the ability of the average man to understand it, but what is vastly more important, it has proved that the work CAN be learned from the book alone by anyone of average intelligence who will apply himself to the task.

This was the authors' fondest hope, their greatest wish, their sincere intention in that writing. The whole world is sick and sinking in a sea of suffering. Almost universally we see around us people who have no other thought than that it is necessary to approach and finally reach an early death through suffering and that to teach a better way is, vaguely, almost a violation of good morals and citizenship and in some cases even sacrilegious. In spite of that, the better way herein taught is so much more desirable, is in reality such good citizenship and such good religion that the authors eagerly grasp the opportunity by the addition of this appendix to make this work even more understandable, so that when and if it becomes necessary to come to death, one can make that approach through a life which has been filled with the joy of living and added years of maximum usefulness.

In 1929 when Section One technic was being organized for teaching, it was realized that here was a mechanical method of healing that the layman could learn and use, and it was determined at that time to set aside this work for the layman. The development of other and more advanced technical works, which with Section One were for the use of the professionals, was continued. But from the use by the layman of the technic contained in this book and as a result of the authors' experience with their own patients, it was demonstrated that under this method health can be restored more rapidly and to a greater degree than under any other previous method. This naturally should create a demand for professionals who would devote all of their time to Aquarian-Age Healing. Therefore, in 1930 in order to meet the demand that it was felt would arise, the teaching of the professionals was commenced. After spending five years in this effort, the results obtained with the professionals have been very unsatisfactory, because they awakened early and rapidly to the fact that a wide-spread knowledge of this system would render their past methods obsolete. This aroused antagonism and a fear that their identity with their own particular school of thought and practice would be lost. Rather than see their less effective methods wholly discarded eventually, the general course of action on their part has taken the form of attempting to absorb into their work such part or parts of Aquarian-Age Healing as best suited their purposes, to the great detriment of this new healing science and the public in general, and depriving the patient of the full benefit to be realized from the exclusive and proper use of this system.

In order to make this work available to all, the first class instruction of laymen began in 1931, as by that time many in the chiropractic profession were equipped to be of assistance should help be desired in the conduct of Section One, as mentioned in Chapter XV. The professionals refused to cooperate. For that reason the whole plan has been practically abandoned, the more easily as it has been discovered that the average layman, after having received instruction, is so far the superior of the professional as a technician that there is no real comparison. The actual fact is that instead of requiring the help of the professional the layman has amply and repeatedly demonstrated his ability to secure betterment and cure in the same cases where the professional has previously failed completely.

Putting all of this together, the professionals have awakened to the fact that they must choose one of two paths and follow the chosen one with every power they have. Either they must destroy this work or some or most of its value and include the balance in their methods, denuded of its identity, hidden in a mass of other material and method and reduced in potency and virtue, or renounce forever former methods and accept this work in toto. This first course of action is the end sought by certain professionals and imitators and which, to some extent, is being accomplished for their own selfish interest. If imitation is the surest measure of success, as has often been said, then Aquarian-Age Healing has given ample proof of its success, even by this measure, as shown by the number and importance of its imitators.

Aquarian-Age Healing, when used in its pure form, restores health so rapidly that some of our professional students have written that they "cannot afford" for this reason to use this method in their practice. Those few professionals who do use it, even passably well, have a larger group of patients than they can comfortably handle, with new ones constantly clamoring to get in, and this without any advertising other than the enthusiasm of their patients.

In this book and appendix, together with other writings by the authors, there is presented the original and only authoritative teaching of Section One technic of Aquarian-Age Healing, and from which all imitators have taken their versions. Their very number, persistence, and diversity are evidences of value that is most easily recognized by the person who is still untaught in its principle. The thought to be gained from this is to make this value your own. False teaching and imitations use technics that employ force and in general are concerned in pushing the vertebrae forward, or anteriorly, further damaging equilibrium. On the other hand, Aquarian-Age Healing regards the vertebrae as merely details in distortion and enables them to regain their natural positions. It allows the body to restore the normal relationships of these and all other parts, thereby establishing equilibrium. All of this is done without forcing the body to do anything. Aquarian-Age

Healing has no antecedents nor was there anything similar to it until after the teaching and publication of its methods.

Medicine, osteopathy, and chiropractic all started out with only a small group of ideas which were added to, changed, modified, and revised over a period of years, so that various schools of thought arose in each group. As a result, no two doctors of the same school, or even from the same institution, will agree in every detail to the same diagnosis or treatment. None of these schools has a more settled form or process than when first introduced. Each is still trying new and discarding previously accepted methods and modalities almost daily. In contrast, there is presented in Aquarian-Age Healing a system complete in almost every detail, with basic principles clearly defined and operative and which can never change. It is a system not founded on mere theories, but one which leaves no room for question or doubt as to what must be done or how.

There are several ways to make a new method of healing well known. The first in the field were the allopaths with practically no competition. In those days the student first spent some time "reading medicine" in the office of someone already practicing and, meantime, performed all the minor tasks for the practitioner. Later, the student was permitted to accompany the professional in his various activities and, finally, upon occasions was entrusted with the actual conduct of various cases. If the student was successful in these, he immediately set himself up as a professional in his own right to continue the practice. It was entirely within his own judgment whether or not he ever took or received any other training of any sort. If he decided that he did desire more training, then at some later date he went to some center where "lecture courses" were given and thus acquired his whole knowledge of the work in which he was engaged.

Then came the homeopaths, the eclectics, the osteopaths, and the chiropractors, to name only the more important ones, who, having made their discoveries, organized their teachings and began very short courses of instruction and turned out their students to practice on the public. The allopaths, in the effort to keep the field clear for themselves, increased their power by legal means and through various legislative enactments, gave more elaborate courses of study, and made a more rigid selection of individuals. They recognized only themselves and through their assumed police powers caused the arrest of all others possible for "practicing medicine without a license."

But the inherent value in other methods of healing and the comparison of their results with the allopathic standards allowed these new entrants into the field to grow in spite of this active antagonism. Now, these groups have each consolidated themselves as securely as possible and in turn emulate the allopaths through what police powers they have been able to gather and add their weight to that of the allopaths in stopping any and all new principles and developments in healing outside of their own ranks.

Aquarian-Age Healing could proceed in this same way, namely, graduate students from a short course and encourage their practice upon the public. Such a mode would be highly profitable because, as such graduates start practicing, all the earlier groups immediately attempt to shut off the new competition by resorting to legal devices, prosecutions, fines, and jail terms for the persons attempting to establish the new system. However, all this attracts public attention, and new students flock into the new schools so that the field of influence rapidly expands in spite of persecution, and finally the public comes to identify it as such. When this happens, then of course new legislation is passed, and the new competitor is now admitted to the august family of the professions.

During all of this time the schools are unmolested, for there is a constitutional guarantee of the right of free speech, of liberty which includes free instruction, and the pursuit of happiness in any way that one pleases, so long as that way does not jeopardize public health, safety, or morals.

But this sort of procedure gives rise to activities on the part of the graduates that are considered to be illegal under our present license system – which, by the way, may some day be proved to be itself illegal. (If you are interested in knowing more of this, send for the authors' free pamphlet on this subject.) Therefore, the authors have refused to engage in such a course of action, even though they could have profited enormously through it. Instead, they have selected a strictly legal method of carrying on the battle for recognition and the right to turn out skilled technicians worthy to compete with any professional of any school. In the meantime, their books and classes are made available to all. They teach by various settled courses of instruction all who desire additional information. Later, as the requirements are better detailed, a professional course will be organized with a training period which, instead of producing graduates in a short time as has always been done before, will be full time and will thoroughly educate students in all necessary sciences, with a background including all these older methods, as well as in Aquarian-Age Healing. All this will come in the due course of events.

This program for expansion and fight for recognition have required and will require that the heaviest and greatest burdens be carried by the founders and originators of Aquarian-Age Healing, but this will save the early graduates from the prosecution and persecution that have so thickly strewn the path of all past modes. It is believed that this program should, by its very *rightness*, attract and keep your support. It should cause you to assist in the suppression of the imitators referred to, as and when they invade the duly protected rights of the discoverers and authors of this work. More than all, it should make you additionally eager to get this work into the hands and thought of all for the general good.

If you had a machine that was capable of turning out sixty pieces an hour without strain and injury and you had great need for the product but the machine operated at only about twenty-five percent of normal, you would not rest until you had it functioning on the highest level of efficiency of the material and structure. Your body and the bodies of those about you have a certain mechanical structure, which when properly alined will function harmoniously and on such a high level of efficiency and ease that it will startle you. How can you rest, knowing that your own body is functioning on a level far below that of which it is capable? The reason that you are not obtaining the full functioning of your material and structure is because your body has sustained some load or loads that exceeded the ability of your body to carry; it is now out of alinement.[17] This prevents your body from resting so you are constantly slowing down. This year you are older than you were last year in efficiency, appearance, and feeling.

This is wrong and unnecessary. A thorough test of Aquarian-Age Healing will prove it to you. Experience this work – have your distortion decreased – and see how much better you work, how much less fatigue you feel, and find to your amazement that at the end of the coming year you not only feel years younger but *look* years younger. This is possible because old age is nothing but accumulated fatigue. By reducing your distortion you eliminate fatigue, and instead of accumulating it you remove the cause for its accumulation. As a result you become healthier and younger in every way and in exact proportion.

A perfectly symmetrical body is a beautiful one. It allows perfect circulation, clear, healthy skin, smooth action, and perfect coordination and control. We expect similar things in our man-made machines. Are we not greater than these?

---

[17] The term *alinement* supersedes the chiropractic term *adjustment* as used in the original *Book One* and is used interchangeably with *Bio-Mechanics* and *Section One*.

Face this thing squarely. Recognize that things worth having must be worked for. Face the responsibilities that this work places upon you; go about it intelligently; do it as set forth; and know the inimitable pleasure that is possible only when you have done a difficult job with true artistry and skill.

This work is difficult for only a short time – which is the time it takes to learn it. One does not learn to drive an automobile efficiently or safely the first time he tries. It takes some practice to make a competent driver. Likewise, it takes practice to become a skilled technician in this work. True, you are working on a human form and that brings increased responsibilities. But when you are driving an automobile, you are also accepting responsibility for human lives.

Because of these responsibilities, you are taken carefully along the path, step by step, but warned of each danger that might arise. It appears that in this endeavor to guard each step so that each student could travel the path with only benefit to the subject, the authors have been misunderstood and that this presentation in *Book One* has caused many readers to hesitate to try the work. This is unwarranted, as has been found by those who have understood the reasons for the warnings, have heeded the sign posts, and with their help have traveled the path and developed a new skill, one of the most valuable of all.

Take these warnings as they were intended. Take each step as it is given, and the knowledge and skill which you will develop will be of such value to you that you would not exchange it for money, because perfect health and the knowledge of how to attain it cannot be measured in dollars.

If you can read and have the use of your arms and fingers, you can learn and use this work. You can build up the health of every member of your family to the point where their resistance is so great that they will not be subject to contagious diseases or to disease of any nature. Thus you can do away with worry over their well-being and save tremendous sums. But the joy of seeing and having beautiful symmetrical, strong, and resistant bodies about you is sufficient reward.

Set aside a certain period each day to be devoted to the study and practice of this work. You cannot afford to put it off, for without health and strength one cannot earn even his daily bread. Distortion saps this strength day by day. Have your distortion corrected and you will build up a strength that will be more than sufficient for your daily labors. Then you will have ample energy stored up and available to support you under some heavier stress that may occur.

Make this book and its teaching a part of your habitual thought processes until you no longer think first of some drug or medicine at the first sign of illness. Learn its procedures so thoroughly that you will never have to even stop and think about just what should be done. Remember that every detail included is there for a very necessary reason and every move that could be safely eliminated is not even mentioned. If you will do this and have the work correctly used on yourself, then as your body comes into alinement you will find the stopping of pain, the cure of acute disease, the correction of your chronic troubles, and the growing of a new and better body than you have ever had, possessing powers that you had thought lost forever – all as the inevitable result and reward of your effort.

The number of cases on which you cannot use this Section One technic is surprisingly small. They consist of those who are unable to stand on their own two feet and cases of severe injury through violence. In injuries through violence, after they have recovered sufficiently to stand up, be sure to work on them. Violence will always drive the center of gravity from its normal position and increase distortion. The only way the person can ever be restored in health and function and through which the effects of violence can be erased is to have the distortion corrected, and this can be done by Section One technic as soon as the person can stand.

This technic, when properly done, will avoid practically every operation that can be done for the so-called betterment of your general health. The only reason for such operations is because the doctor is unable to restore function and health to the part. An organ so removed is irretrievably lost. Re-alining the body *will* restore function and health to the part as well as to the whole – *will* save you the dangers of anesthesia and of being left with a permanently crippled mechanism.

After you have saved a few friends from operations and have yourself been so preserved, you will truly value the fact that you do not need constantly to call on the doctor. You will have proven that you can do more than he.

All of these things are in your own hands at this moment as you read this book. Because that is so and is a simple, actual fact, this one more statement is warranted:

THIS IS THE MOST IMPORTANT BOOK THAT HAS EVER BEEN WRITTEN ON THE SUBJECT OF HEALTH OR THE CARE OF THE BODY OR THE CURE OF DISEASE.

Doubt that if you will, but for your own good and for the good of your loved ones, do not pass this book by without proving that you really have done what the best of doctors have failed to do for you and them in the past and that you are in better health than you thought possible for you. YOU CAN DO IT.

In passing now to the details of the technic, included here with only minor changes from the bulletin, please refer to the pages noted in the book proper and make the applications as they appear.

On page 169 in the book in numbers 4, 5, and 7, we use the word "adjust." This has led to some misunderstanding, and to clarify, these paragraphs should read:

4. The effect of the contact is principally through the center of gravity via the sacrum and secondarily on every bone, muscle, and functioning tissue in the body. As the sacrum is the structural center of the body and holds all other parts in

correct or incorrect relationships through muscles originating from it, directly or indirectly, we need concern ourselves with the position of the sacrum only. The correct or incorrect position of all other parts of the body, correct or incorrect posture, is an indication of the correct or incorrect position of the sacrum. Any work done on the other parts of the body for the purpose of alining it almost invariably moves this structural center further from normal and, therefore, is detrimental from the standpoint of health.

5. We never move any sacrum except from the *inferior* and *anterior*, the direction being slightly superior and mostly posterior.

7. In Section One technic we never take contact directly on the sacrum, but use the soft tissue to influence the sacrum correctly. Only the posterior surface of the sacrum is presented to the worker, and no contact on this surface can bring it backwards.

We add some notes in explanation of the "line of direction" and "line of pull."[18] The body must be brought back and into its proper gravity line, and under no consideration can you bring it too far backwards. Get all of that effect you can, both in the standing and bench contacts. Do not push at all, and especially not headwards nor toward the front of the body *in any case*, but always try to get the body and the anterior buttock to come as far *backwards* as it is possible. If you use too heavy a contact on the backward pull you will unbalance your patient, produce resistance and contracture, and increase the distortion. The contact is a gentle urging of the body back into

---

[18] *Line of drive, line of direction,* and *line of force* are used interchangeably in reference to the *secondary line of direction. Line of pull* refers to the *primary line of direction (drive).* Instructions regarding these were clarified and updated significantly in Dr. Hurley's later classes, including the concept of *vectors* and methods for *proving the contact.*

line. Wait for the body to respond of itself – do not try to pull it.

When you are advised to use only as much force at the end of the work as would slightly spatter a ripe cranberry, it means that if you are wrong or not exactly right, you will find that it is actually not at all possible to do anything much more than just "slip off" the contact. The fact is that the contact must be directed usually so far *backwards* in order to get all the soreness and pain out of the points marked that sometimes it is next to impossible to hold onto it at all. So if at first you are unable to maintain the point chosen, that is a sign that you are actually progressing with due care and judgment and that in due time you will develop a high degree of skill and get the most gratifying results. Even if it should be that you cannot hold the contact long enough to clear all the sore spots, do not be discouraged. Take contact again in exactly the right spot and in exactly the right way and continue the alinement.

If you are unable to eliminate completely all the sore spots the first time you try, do not let that disturb you, for even a small attempt, if done as is taught, will make some minor changes which will assist you in the next alinement. These changes will improve the patient so much that it will seem incredible that such a "little thing" can be responsible for the changes which will occur and be noticed.

Though it is possible, as mentioned in the text of the book, to work all day if need be in a severe case, yet in the average case under a skilled technician, thirty minutes from the first step to the last step gives the best results. Various people have been given a single thirty-minute alinement, followed by no other work or attention of any sort, and it has been found that there are definite and continuing results covering a period of not hours or days merely, but in one case for at least three years afterwards. In another case in which there was a bad curvature of the spine, the patient so straightened up from one such alinement that he became five and a quarter inches taller in the period of five weeks following it, while attending to all of the ordinary affairs of a chicken farm and without any other attention of any sort.

Many cases of acute diseases have been completely cured by one such alinement. Even chronic conditions such as hernias, in special cases, have been cured by one such alinement, while other cases of different types but of the same disease require much longer time and much more work. It all depends upon the rapidity with which the distortion can be reduced. So do not be discouraged by slow results, nor on the other hand do not be surprised at seeming miracles, nor believe that the alinement was effective in the one case and not in the other. The difference is in the responsiveness and in the vital power of the patient, if we assume that the work was equally good in each case. This can always be seen and measured by noting the rapid or slow improvement in the distortion of the subject.

Remember, this work is not primarily a treatment of symptoms, though it will correct every one of them in the most rapid and best way, but it is essentially a method, and the only natural one ever conceived, for the correction of *disease itself.* The body will take care of the process and each of the processes in their turn and in their proper order, doing the things that are the most essential for the continued life and return to health first, and attending to the other matters in their order. You neither can nor should have any concern about that, for no one, not even the most learned or skilled doctor, knows even a small part of the things that would have to be known to make this interference intelligent or helpful.

This technic may be used under the roughest and most trying circumstances – for instance, in the mountains using a rock-weighted string tied to a tree limb for lining up your patient and determining contact. The ground or a log may serve as a work bench.

But when you are working regularly in your own home on your family, the following suggestions regarding equipment will be found to make the work easier for both you and your patient.[19]

Secure a piece of laminated wood 15" x 28" in size and a 3/8" strip of wood or metal 28" long to be fastened down the center of the board. Then have two additional strips 7 5/16" long to be fastened on either side of the center strip at right angles to it and 12 inches from the back end. Put a screw eye in the center strip on the extreme back end. The feet are placed one on either side of the center strip, as closely as possible, the instep over the right angle strip with the front of the heel pressed close to it. This allows an easier and more accurate placing of the feet.

Plan where you can place your foot board so that it will be disturbed the least. In putting up your plumb line, a wire can be fastened from the picture moulding on one side of the wall to the moulding on the opposite side. Then drop a plumb line down from the moulding where the wire is fastened and fasten same to the base board of your room. Be sure this line is plumb. Place the center of the 28" strip on the foot board up to this plumb line.

Next drop a plumb line from the wire down to the screw eye at the back of the foot board. Be sure it is plumb. If a light spring is used between the wire and string, the line will remain taut. Your patient stands in front of the plumb line fastened on the back of the foot board, facing the plumb line that drops down the wall.

When you stand behind your patient, close one eye and sight over the one string to the other. When these are in direct line, then you will know you are directly behind your patient and in a position to make correct measurements.

The bench or table should be about six feet long and about 24 inches high, measured from the floor to the under-surface of the table, as it is more comfortable for the operator to be

---

[19] Dr. Hurley later simplified and improved the instructions regarding the foot board (T-square), plumb line, and therapy table.

seated. The table should be sufficiently narrow toward the head end – from 12 to 14 inches – to allow the patient's arms to drop over the sides, hands resting on a small shelf attached to the front legs about 15 inches from the floor. Cut a rectangular hole in the head end and do not pad. Begin your padding about 12 inches from the head end. Then use a small soft pillow with an elongated opening to support the face. In this way the patient's head is not raised above the level of the body. Then you will need a firm roll to go under the patient's hips and another for his ankles so his body can be quite relaxed and comfortable.

Make and date a sketch of each patient similar to the one on page 166 so that improvement can be noted. Remember that you observe the departure from the perpendicular line by noting the midpoint of the patient's swaying. Remember also that if you should get the wrong contact and bad results, you should go back to the beginning, placing the patient in front of the string, eyes closed and body as relaxed as possible, and check up for the proper anteriority and degree of departure from the string line before proceeding.

Having made and recorded your findings, then refer to the position of the line between the buttocks in relation to the string, and mark its deviation from normal in inches or fractions of inches on your diagram, for this deviation, along with the anterior buttock, determines the point of contact. In the illustrations, all cases shown have the line between the buttocks parallel with the string line. In cases where the line between the buttocks slants toward or away from the string line, note the amount of deviation at the top of the line as well as at the bottom of this line, and use the top measurement to determine the point of contact and direction.

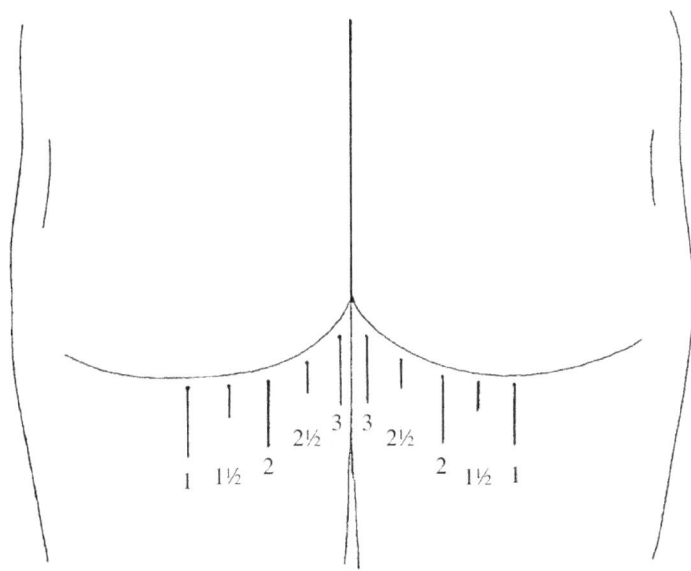

Figure 15 – Points of Contact

You will note in Figure 15 that the furthest laterally for the point of contact as taken on the buttock is one-half the width of the thigh as measured just below the buttock. This is because we are working on the center of gravity of the body by means of the sacrum through the gluteus maximus muscle. In contacting this muscle from the point corresponding with the middle of the thigh or nearer to the median line, we confine the contact to those fibers of the gluteus maximus muscle that arise from the sacrum only. Do not take contact any further to the outside than point one.

There are five possible points of contact on each buttock to be discussed. Only *one* of these is the best one for any distortion presented. A different point may be indicated when the distortion is changed as a result of alinements. These points are illustrated in Figure 15.

The point on the buttock that corresponds to the middle of the thigh is designated for convenience as contact point number one, as this corrects the simplest type of distortion, as

explained on page 169. The point on the buttock that
corresponds to the postero-median border of the thigh is
designated as point number three, and the point that falls
midway between point number one and point number three is
designated as point number two. Do not change the position of
your eye after marking number one, but mark all divisions as
they look from here, just as illustrated.

An eyebrow pencil may be used for marking the body. Make
all marks very gently so as not to increase distortion. It is very
strongly advised that these points be marked *on the thigh* in
every case before the standing contact is even attempted, as it
guides the operator to the proper point both in the standing
contact as well as in the bench contact. After placing these
marks on the thigh, you will note that there is still room for a
contact point between number one and number two; also room
for another contact point between number two and number
three. So these points are also marked and are designated as
number one and one-half and number two and one-half, as
shown in Figure 15.

CONTACT IS ALWAYS TAKEN ON THE ANTERIOR
BUTTOCK, as explained on page 168, and the original anterior
buttock is considered the anterior buttock except as noted on
page 182. The anteriority is measured on the level of the most
prominent part of the buttocks, which is down toward the
thigh, and record is made of this by marking the letter "A" on
the drawing of the case on the proper side.

Now for the line of direction to be used from these points of
contact and HOW TO DETERMINE WHICH POINT IS THE
CORRECT ONE TO USE.

From any determined point of contact, various directions of
pull are indicated, as shown by the illustrations in Figure 16.
This direction remains constant and must be considered and
held at all times while clearing tender spots. It is a gentle
backward pull away from the patient's body. *This* direction is
approximately at right angles to the vertical line when used in

the standing contact, and the only variation in the direction of pull depends upon the different degrees of sagging found in different buttocks. Call this the "Primary Line of Direction." The contact includes a gentle urging of the body in a posterior direction when the patient is standing and in a direction up away from the body when the patient is on the bench.

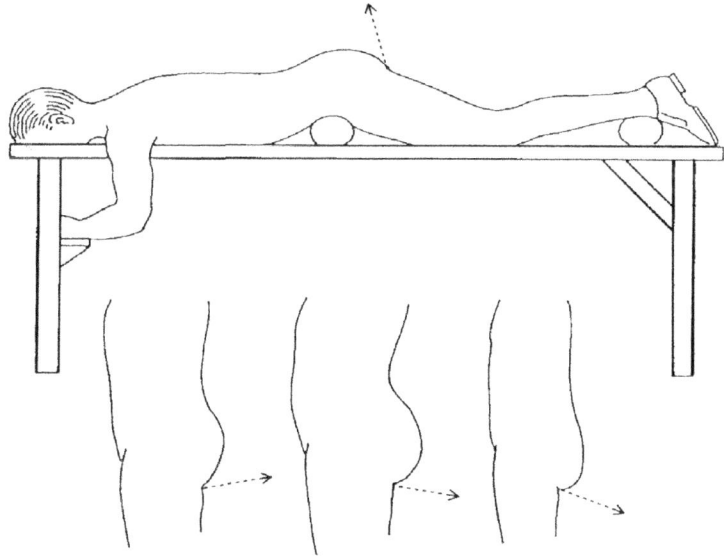

Figure 16 – Primary Line of Direction or Backward Pull

Figures 17 to 21, inclusive, show the difference in the lines of direction which may be necessary in order to correct the abnormal departures of the body shown by the back of the patient in relation to the string line, that is, the side to side and rotational distortion.

In other words, the technician must observe two directions: the one above discussed and shown in Figure 16, and the one indicated on Figures 17 to 21, inclusive, which we shall call the "Secondary Line of Direction."

After standing contact is taken and held long enough to prove its correctness – without moving the contact finger and while still holding contact and direction, gently outline with the eyebrow pencil the upper part of the finger on the buttock. Still holding the same gentle, accurate contact, draw a line upward from this outline indicating the secondary line of direction of the contact.

RULES FOR DETERMINING SECONDARY LINE OF DIRECTION (Figures 17-21, Inclusive)

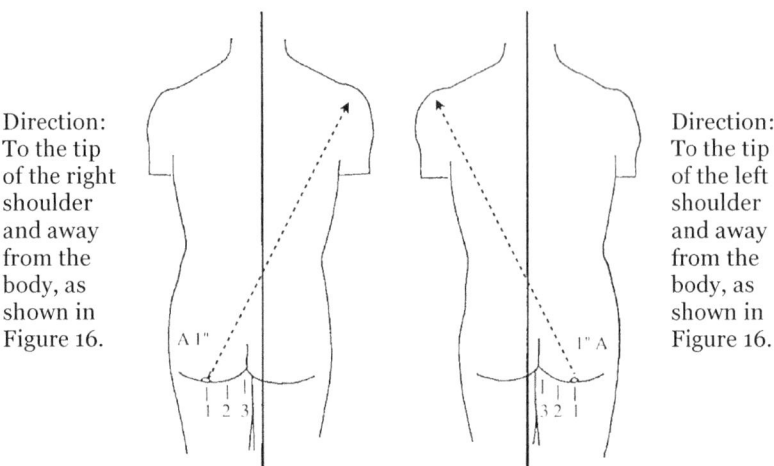

Direction: To the tip of the right shoulder and away from the body, as shown in Figure 16.

Direction: To the tip of the left shoulder and away from the body, as shown in Figure 16.

Figure 17 – Point One Contact and Direction

POINT ONE CONTACT is taken on the anterior buttock when the line between the buttocks is one inch or more over on the same side of the string as the anterior buttock, that is, when the string line does *not* pass the buttock which is to be used for contact. The secondary line of direction is to the tip of the opposite shoulder as shown in Figure 17, remembering as always that the primary line of direction is to the *posterior* and only *slightly superior*, just enough to allow the holding of contact.

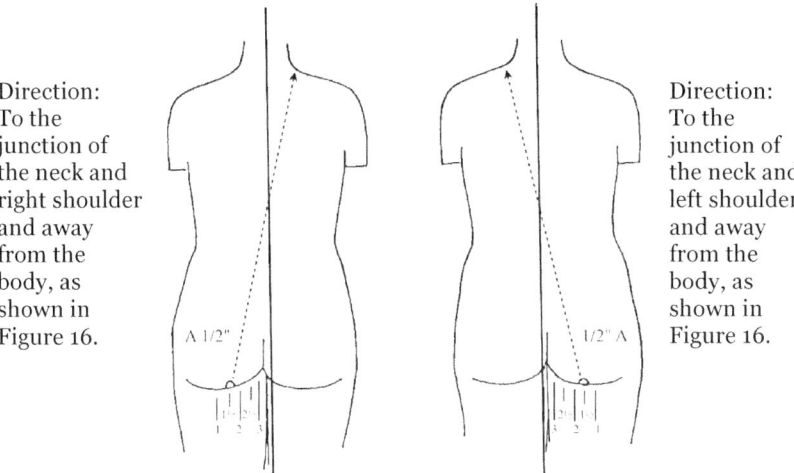

Direction: To the junction of the neck and right shoulder and away from the body, as shown in Figure 16.

Direction: To the junction of the neck and left shoulder and away from the body, as shown in Figure 16.

Figure 18 – Point One and One-Half Contact and Direction

POINT ONE AND ONE-HALF CONTACT is taken when the line between the buttocks is approximately one-half inch over on the same side of the string as the anterior buttock, that is, when the string line does *not* pass the buttock that is to be used for contact. The secondary line of direction is to the junction of the neck and shoulder of the opposite side, as shown in Figure 18, and away from the body, as shown in Figure 16.

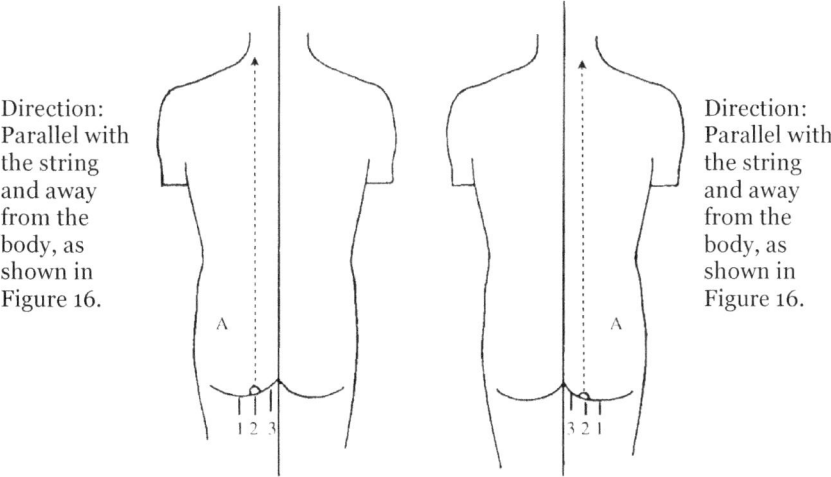

Direction: Parallel with the string and away from the body, as shown in Figure 16.

Direction: Parallel with the string and away from the body, as shown in Figure 16.

Figure 19 – Point Two Contact and Direction

POINT TWO CONTACT is taken when the line between the buttocks is "on" the string or very nearly so, that is, one-fourth inch or less away from the string line. The contact is taken, as always, on the anterior buttock. The secondary line of direction is parallel with the string line, as shown in Figure 19, and away from the body, as shown in Figure 16.

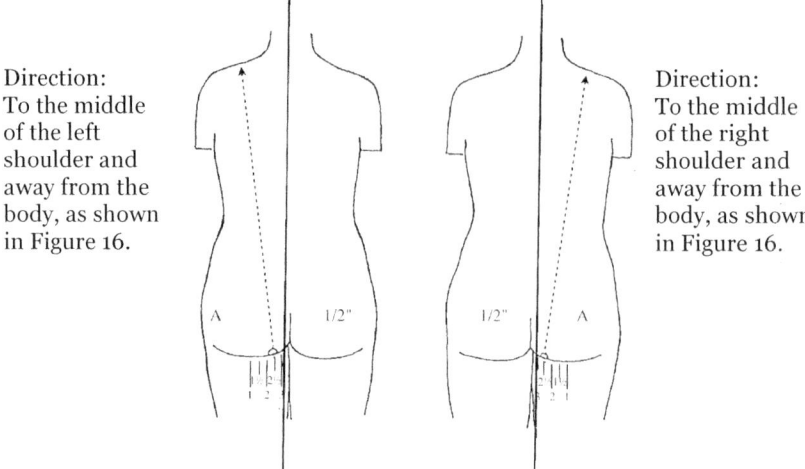

Direction: To the middle of the left shoulder and away from the body, as shown in Figure 16.

Direction: To the middle of the right shoulder and away from the body, as shown in Figure 16.

Figure 20 – Point Two and One-Half Contact and Direction

POINT TWO AND ONE-HALF CONTACT is taken when the line between the buttocks is approximately one-half inch over on the side of the string opposite the anterior buttock, that is, when the line of the string *does* pass the buttock which is to be used for contact, as shown in Figure 20. The secondary line of direction is to the middle of the shoulder on the *same* side as the anterior buttock, and away from the body, as shown in Figure 16.

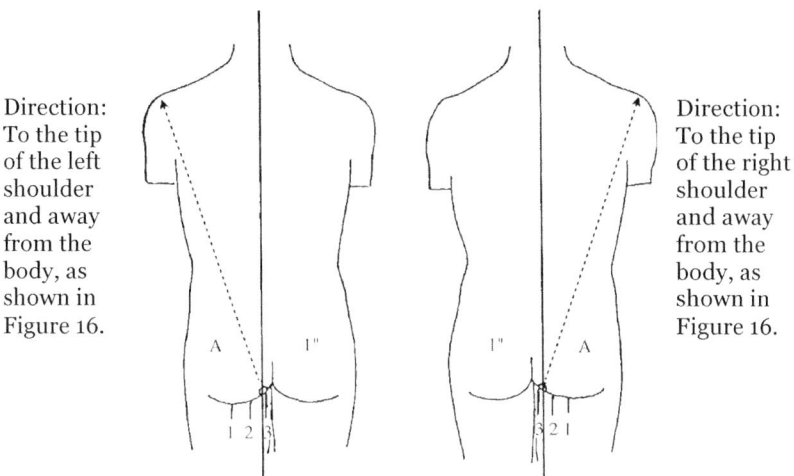

Direction: To the tip of the left shoulder and away from the body, as shown in Figure 16.

Direction: To the tip of the right shoulder and away from the body, as shown in Figure 16.

Figure 21 – Point Three Contact and Direction

POINT THREE CONTACT is taken when the line between the buttocks is one inch or more over on the side of the string opposite the anterior buttock, that is, when the line of the string *does* pass the buttock which is to be used for contact, as shown in Figure 21.

The secondary line of direction is to the tip of the shoulder on the *same* side as the anterior buttock, and away from the body, as shown in Figure 16.

If these rules are accurately followed, along with all of those in the body of the book, good results can be expected in every patient who is able to stand so that you can measure distortion. It is important to record the relation of the line between the buttocks with the line between the thighs, as well as all those others given on the chart on page 166. These findings are not used in the determination of the point of contact, but as a check for progress in the elimination of distortion.

This appendix does not change any rule written in the body of the book nor alter any except as herein stated. This method of locating contact, herein given to you, is exact and correct in all cases. It has been used in this teaching for a period of five years. There is at least one other method equally efficient, but not so easy to reduce to simple written rule, and therefore you are urged to confine all of your work to these particular points, governed by this particular method.

Having performed all the above, having seen favorable response on the part of the patient, having made your marks on the buttock, you are now ready to place the patient on the bench, where you will proceed as before instructed.

Having now marked all the sore, tender, or numb areas, and taken contact as nearly as possible as you did when the patient was standing, being guided by the mark on the buttock, you now proceed to clear the complained-of areas. Very occasionally it happens that they are all gone as a result of one alinement. The fact that these tender spots clear under the first alinement does not mean that the patient is now free from distortion. You have taken away enough distortion to allow the relaxation of some superficial contractures. The next time you work on that patient you will be able to eliminate some of the deeper trouble. This will explain why some tender areas permanently disappear and new areas are brought to the surface. As the distortion is decreased, the patient becomes more responsive with fewer tender areas to clear.

Never change the point of contact at all during a single alinement and never change the secondary line of direction so greatly that it would overlap the line from any other contact point. Confine yourself to these limits, for perfection lies within them. Then slowly, carefully, with understanding and definite objective, strive to find the EXACT direction from that point of contact that will perfectly clear every one of the marked sore areas. It can be done. You can do it. Here is the difference between skill and the lack of it. Here is the test of your work and understanding. Be guided exclusively by these instructions and the book itself, and you will, even if you fail to complete the job, do a vast amount of good and prepare the way for complete success in the future.

After having cleared all of the tender and numb areas, always place your patient in front of the string and check for progress made, noting the changes in the patient's body. Do this both for your own satisfaction and for the building up of confidence in your own work and ability. Since the publication of *Book One*, it has been found that it is not necessary to have the patient rest first for one-half an hour, as mentioned on page 181. In some cases where the patient feels the need of resting, you can advise him to do so after you have completed the alinement. Until some skill is developed, it is better not to attempt alinements of very young children nor of those persons who are very ill.

If you should try this work and then feel that you are in need of additional instruction, that too is available. The founders of Aquarian-Age Healing at present are operating correspondence courses, as well as personal instruction classes. These correspondence courses did, in the first year of their operation, set a standard previously unheard of in the whole past history of such instruction. Statistics show that less than ten percent of correspondence courses in general are ever completed. This figure embraces all schools and all sorts of courses.

Courses in Aquarian-Age Healing have to date been completed by everyone who has ever enrolled, or they are in process of completion at the moment. It has never in any instance even been necessary to suggest that the work should not be allowed to drag. Every student has done the work as rapidly as possible, and every student has acquired a technic that is productive, to say nothing of less direct benefits. The authors are proud of this record and invite your further inquiry.

Each course is available at a very reasonable price. In addition, there is in the near future a professional course to be offered, and the mastery of the work taught in this book will be one of the necessary entrance requirements. Information concerning all of this and concerning the advanced technics and the further developments of principle concerned in this work, which constitute the professional sections, can be obtained upon request from the Headquarters Office in Fort Lauderdale. Address all communications regarding this work or instruction in it to Aquarian-Age Healing Institute, Ft. Lauderdale, Fla., International Headquarters, Dr. John L. Hurley, Founder, Director.[20]

---

[20] This is no longer an active address.

GLOSSARY

Note: Dr. Hurley's later developments and revisions are outside the scope of this publication. (See Foreword.) However, to add clarification and aid understanding of concepts in Book One, a glossary of terms and definitions that he used in his later classes is included here.

Acidosis is the term used to describe the condition of the body when acids accumulate abnormally and produce disturbances that are noticeable.

Adaptation is that new relation of structure which best permits function in an abnormal condition.

Aquarian-Age Healing relates to everything in the universe. It is the study of distortion, its causes, its effects, and the means for its correction. **Bio-Mechanics** and **Bio-Engineering** are its reduction of principle to accurate statement and technic.

Center of Gravity is that point of any structure from which it can be supported and will not tip, tilt, roll, or slide.

Deflection is that departure from previous form under loading which is completely, immediately, and automatically corrected by removal of the load. Deflection is caused by stress.

Deform means damage in form, decreased usefulness.

Deformity should be used exclusively in relation to living process, and there to mean growth into a distorted pattern.

Distort is to twist into some shape not previously held.

Distortion is that departure from previous form under loading which is not completely, immediately, and automatically corrected by removal of the load. Distortion is caused by strain.

Elastic limit is the name of the iso point where stress becomes strain.

Evolution is a process of orderly and gradual change or development.

Form is that which denotes usefulness.

Hurley's Syllogism:

Exhaustion is the only cause of death.

Fatigue is some degree of exhaustion.

Degrees and amounts of fatigue measure the approach of exhaustion.

Disease is some degree of death.

Degrees and amounts of disease measure the approach of death.

Exhaustion	=	**Death**
Fatigue	=	**Disease**
Rest	=	**Cure**

Iso point is that point at which a change of state occurs.

Pain is nature's warning of damage being done.

Rest is a state of slight muscular tonus which maintains the body's shape, condition for function, and readiness for near-instant response at all times, with a minimum amount of lactic acid formed and entirely eliminated.

Strain is the name of the internal condition of any structure under any load which exceeds the elastic limit of that structure. Strain is destructive.

Stress is the name of the internal condition of any structure under any load which does not exceed the elastic limit of that structure. Stress is constructive.

Torque means to twist.

INDEX

Note: *In cases where a particular entry is discussed on two or more continuous pages, only the first page number is given.*

ABOUT THE AUTHORS

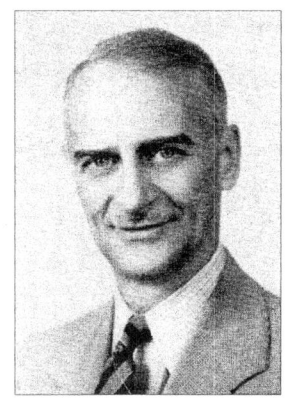

John L. Hurley was born in 1883 in Pennsylvania. Following a successful career as a mechanical engineer, he became a chiropractor in 1914. Combining his knowledge of mechanical engineering principles and human physiology, he developed the essential principles and technics of a new system of manual therapy, which he named Aquarian-Age Healing. After publishing two books with co-author Helen Sanders in the early 1930s, Dr. Hurley devoted his life to practicing, improving, and teaching Aquarian-Age Healing.

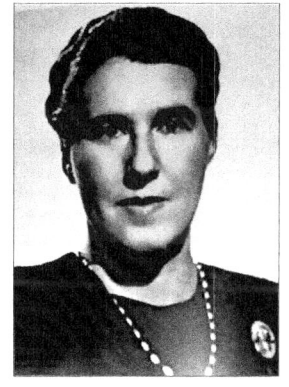

Helen Sanders was born in California in 1903 and graduated from Los Angeles Chiropractic College in 1929. In 1930 she joined Dr. Hurley to establish the firm Hurley and Sanders in Los Angeles, and they were married from 1931 to 1937. Dr. Sanders held an active chiropractic license throughout her long career and was highly respected in the field. From 1949 to 1962, she was the owner and president of the Hollywood Chiropractic College, which was attended by many students who would become prominent leaders in the chiropractic profession.

Ken Ladd and Shay O'Neal were students of the late Dr. E.F. Hayles, who was one of Dr. Hurley's last students. They were also mentored by another of Dr. Hurley's last students, the late Dr. John H. Tomlinson. Dr. Hayles and Dr. Tomlinson were practitioners of Aquarian-Age Healing for over forty-five years. In 1991 Dr. Hayles, as director of the Aquarian-Age Healing Institute, certified Ken Ladd to teach basic and advanced levels of Aquarian-Age Healing.

www.bionomicshealthinstitute.com

Printed in Great Britain
by Amazon